30-DAY PALEO CHALLENGE

CHANGE YOUR LIFE AND LOSE 15 POUNDS WITH PALEO DIET

SHANE RIIZ

TABLE OF CONTENTS

INTRODUCTION

In 2014, the World Health Organization (WHO) reported that there are over 1.9 billion adults (18 years and above) who are overweight. Of this number, 600 million individuals are obese. Health experts consider the growing statistics of overweight and obesity as "alarming" since according to WHO, both the conditions are "linked to a lot of deaths worldwide..." Individuals who are overweight and obese have a higher risk of developing health problems such as cardiac ailments, type 2 diabetes, hypertension, high cholesterol levels, stroke, different types of cancer and sleep apnea.

One way to determine whether your weight is normal, overweight, or obese, you can calculate your body mass index or BMI. To compute your BMI take your weight in kilograms and divide it by the square of your height in meters.

For example:

Weight:: 68 kg.

Height: 1.75 m

BMI= $68/(1.75)^2$

22.20

And then use this table below to see whether your BMI range if your weight is ideal, normal, overweight or obese.

BMI	Category
16.5 to 18.5	Underweight
18.5 to 25	Ideal
25 to 30	Overweight
30 to 35	Obese
35 to 40	Clinically Obese
40 and above	Dangerously Obese

If your BMI is 25.0 and above, it means that you're overweight, and you need to do something about it.

Other than your BMI, another indication whether you're at risk of developing the health problems I mentioned above is your belly fat. According to the National Heart, Lung, and Blood Institute (NIH), having fat on your midsection rather than your hips, puts you at a higher risk of developing severe health conditions; and your waist circumference can determine whether you're a candidate or not. Having a waistline of more than 35 inches for women and 40 inches for men puts them at more risk of having heart problems and type 2 diabetes.

Now you're probably wondering, what does the problem of overweight and obesity and its health risks have to do with the Paleo Diet? Well, that's because poor eating habits (diet filled with low nutrition food) is seen as one of the leading causes of overweight and obesity—and the Paleo Diet is the answer to preventing or even reverse being overweight.

Don't worry if you're unfamiliar with Paleo, because this book contains all the information you need to know about the diet. Here's what you will learn in this book:

- The principles of the Paleo Diet
- How the "modern" diet has affected your weight, and how Paleo can counter it's effects
- The health benefits of going Paleo
- Tips on how you can ready yourself from going Paleo
- The foods that you should avoid and stock up on
- Delicious and easy-to-make Paleo recipes you can whip up in your kitchen

I congratulate you for taking the initiative to begin a lifestyle change by buying this book. I hope you'll find this book "30-Day Paleo Challenge: Change Your Life and Lose 15 Pounds with Paleo Diet" helpful as you move towards a healthier version of you!

Now I challenge you to try out the 30-day paleo challenge and see how Paleo can change your life!

Best of luck!

Chapter 1: All You Need to Know About the Paleo Diet

I'm pretty sure that even before you downloaded this book, you've read or heard of the Paleo Diet at least once or twice. Well, that's because the Paleo Diet has gained popularity for being one of the healthiest fitness diets with celebrities, athletes, and other cross-fitters following the principles of Paleo. In fact, Paleo was recognized as the most researched diets on Google in 2013.

What is the Paleo Diet?

Also known as the "Caveman Diet," the Paleo Diet is a nutrient-rich food regimen patterned from the diet of our hunter-gatherer ancestors (cavemen) of the Paleolithic Era. The principle of Paleo is simple: avoid the type of foods which were not available during the Paleolithic Era which means that "modern food" (grains, farm-grown meat, dairy, sweets, processed food, etc.) had been eliminated in the Paleo Diet.

Although Paleo has only been popular in the year 2000's, it was actually in the early 1900s, 1913 to be exact, when Joseph Knowles suggested a healthier diet after a two-month experiment living in the wilderness. Knowles claimed that he became more fit and stronger after living as a hunter-gatherer, like that of our cavemen ancestors.

This idea was followed a few decades after when gastroenterologist, Dr. Walter L. Voegtin coined the term "Paleo Diet" in his book." The Stone Age Diet" which was published in 1975. In his book, Voegtin's suggests that 99.9% of the modern man's genetic code came from our hunter-gatherer ancestors and this means that our bodies naturally survive on the diet like that of our ancestors from the Stone Age.

This idea has also gained the interest of a few scientists and anthropologists who also published research papers about the diet. It was however only in the year 2013 when the Paleo Diet gained immense popularity from the public after nutrition expert Loren Cordain launched the Paleo Diet Movement.

What's wrong with the "Modern Diet"?

As you now know, the basic idea of the Paleo Diet is to avoid all types of food which were not available during the Stone Age. So what's wrong with the "modern diet"?

Simply by comparing the physical state of an average caveman to an average modern-day man, you can already see that cavemen were lean, strong, and agile while the modern man is physically unfit and is sluggish. What could be the reason why man has transitioned from being fit to become overweight?

Proponents of the Paleo Diet believe that the dawn of the Agricultural Age has changed the way man ate. From being meat eaters, men became so dependent on farm-raised foods (grains, pasta, bread, and other carb-rich foods) which were very different from what the cavemen ate. The problem here is that, although man's diet changed, our genetic makeup has not evolved over the last thousands of years, and this means that our bodies are still not accustomed to most of the foods available today.

Farming made us believe that to be the satiated majority of our diet must be made of carbohydrate rich foods. This high-carb diet, however, is seen to be a major contributor as to why man's physique has regressed from being fit to fat. When carbohydrates are consumed, our body transforms them into glucose, which is used as energy. However, when glucose is not burned as energy, it turns into body fat, and this explains why people who live sedentary lifestyles have extra pounds of fat! Physical activities are essential to burn the carbs which you consume.

Processed foods and food servings which come in huge servings are also seen as the primary culprits as to why the statistics of overweight individuals have been ballooning over the decades.

The Paleo Diet works by simply re-programming our diet to what it was originally designed. By eliminating "unnatural foods" such as carb-rich, processed, high fat and sugar laden foods, Paleo can help you to be more fit and strong like our cavemen ancestors.

Benefits of the Paleo Diet

Since the Paleo Diet offers a healthier alternative, here are some of the health benefits you can gain from going Paleo:

1. Enables weight loss — By eating Paleo-approved foods, you eliminate carb-rich, high in fat, and sugar laden foods which contribute to weight gain. You consume more nutritious and fiber-rich foods which enable the body to shed off unwanted weight.

2. Increases energy — Most people think that going on a "diet" means restricting your daily food consumption. In contrary, the Paleo Diet encourages one to eat three nutritious meals a day, even with light snacks in between as long as you stick to the Paleo-approve foods and this means that your body will have enough energy to burn all throughout the day.

3. Builds muscles — Since the Paleo Diet promotes the consumption of meat, your body gets the proper amount of protein it needs to generate and repair muscles. This particular Paleo Diet benefit is perfect for bodybuilders and athletes, who need protein in their diet.

4. Proper digestion — Other than meat, consumption of veggies and fruits are also encouraged in the Paleo Diet. And as you know, fruits and vegetables are a good source of fiber that is essential for proper digestion.

5. Reduces the risk of developing diet-related diseases — Through the Paleo Diet, you can avoid foods (processed food and junk food) that heighten your risk of developing diet-related illnesses like hypertension, stroke and diabetes type 2.

Types of Paleo Diet

There are two types of the Paleo Diet you can follow, the **Restrictive** and the **Less-restrictive** Paleo Diet. As a beginner, I suggest you try the less-restrictive type.

Although the idea of Paleo is to eliminate foods which are not available in the Stone Age, the less restrictive type of Paleo allows you to consume the following:

- o Fruits and vegetable juices- modern Paleos are allowed to consume their fruits and vegetables by using kitchen equipment such as juicers and blenders.

- o Supplements- although cavemen didn't have access to supplements during their time, the modern Paleo are allowed to take vitamins and minerals in the likes of fish oils, protein powders, etc. for their diet.

- o Light processed foods- this is beneficial for people who adhere to Paleo diet and who don't have the time to cook their food from scratch.

- o Wine and Dark Chocolate- Less-restrictive Paleos are allowed to consume wine and dark chocolate (which are considered healthy food) in controlled amounts.

For a more strict Paleo Diet, here are the types of food you should totally avoid:

- o Nightshades- vegetables such as tomatoes, eggplant, hot peppers, etc. should be eliminated in your diet.

- o Starchy vegetables- say goodbye to potatoes, peas, beets, etc. If you already have problems with high sugar levels or are already categorized as obese, then eliminating this type of food will be good for you.

- o No sweeteners— since our ancestors didn't use any sweeteners during their time, sugar and even artificial sweeteners must be avoided (except honey).

If you think you are ready to go Paleo, go on to the next chapter to get started with the Paleo Diet.

Chapter 2: Getting Ready for the Paleo Diet

Learning about the benefits of Paleo would encourage you to follow the diet. However, what I want you to realize that choosing to go Paleo does not mean that you should only follow this diet for an "x" amount of time and then go back to your usual diet after you've reached your weight goal. Going Paleo means that you're choosing to change your lifestyle entirely. If you think you're ready for the challenge, here are some tips you can follow to jumpstart your new found lifestyle.

1. **Consult your health care provider** — Although Paleo is practically a safe and healthy diet, I recommend that you consult your doctor first especially if you already have an existing health condition. Going Paleo means that you're going to eliminate some food types in your meals, and you just might need a go-signal from your doctor before pursuing the diet.

2. **Create goals** — Setting goals are important as you begin your Paleo journey. You can ask yourself these following questions: "Do I want to lose weight?", "Do I want to build muscles?", or "Do I want to improve my stamina?"

   Focus on these goals because these will help you pursue the Paleo lifestyle.

3. **Do your research** — Event though this book will introduce you to the basics of the Paleo Diet, I encourage you to continue learning about this diet. Also, it will be helpful to seek different exercises that complement the Paleo diet hence this will help you achieve your weight goals faster.

4. **Do a pantry clean-up** — Transitioning from your usual diet to a Paleo Diet will be harder for you if you let "temptations" lurk in your pantry. If you want to start the Paleo lifestyle, one of the major step that you need to do it to clean out your pantry. Remove any food that is not Paleo-approved. Say goodbye to the chips, ice cream, dairy, etc.

5. **Go on a shopping trip** — After you've purged out your pantry, the next thing to do is go on a shopping trip. Your goal is to fill your refrigerator

with Paleo-friendly foods. I will give you a comprehensive list of Paleo foods in the next chapter. But the tip I'd like to leave you is to skip on the aisles which will tempt you to buy foods that are not part of the Paleo Diet. Well this will not only prevent you from buying junk and processed foods, but it will also save you time from going through all the aisles in the grocery.

6. **Find a buddy** — Your lifestyle change will be much easier if you have a friend who will support you through your journey. Ask your partner or your friends to try the Paleo Diet with you. Look for someone who will inspire you and will motivate you to keep on pursuing the Paleo lifestyle.

7. **Keep a record** — One way to motivate yourself to keep on going is by keeping a track record of your performance. On the first day of your Paleo journey, I'd like you to journal your weight and your health conditions. As you progress in the Paleo Diet, you will see how far you've come from having extra weight to becoming leaner and fit.

8. **Do it now!** The most important thing that you should do is to DO IT NOW! There's no better time choosing a healthier path than now! If you feel like a lifestyle change seems a little bit daunting, challenge yourself to do a 30-day trial first to see the benefits of the Paleo Diet.

Chapter 3: The Paleo Grocery List for Successfully Losing 15 Pounds

What's great about the Paleo Diet is that even though you're pursuing a healthier diet, it doesn't mean that it limits you to only some food types. In fact, you will realize that Paleo offers a variety of foods which you can enjoy. Here is a comprehensive list (less-restrictive) of Paleo-friendly foods.

1. **Protein** - in choosing which type of meat you should buy, the rule of thumb is to stick to lean foods, naturally or organically grown meats. You can buy frozen meat, but it's best that you stay away from canned goods.

   Meat

   - Chicken meat (preferably breast)
   - Turkey (without skin)
   - Pork chops
   - Lean ground pork or beef
   - Beef flank steak
   - Sirloin steak
   - Eggs

   Fish (almost any type of fish)

   - Salmon
   - Tuna
   - Bass
   - Striped Bass
   - Mackerel
   - Herring
   - Trout
   - Cod
   - Grouper
   - Eel
   - Bluefish
   - Red Snapper

Shell Fish

- o Shrimp
- o Lobster
- o Crab
- o Mussels
- o Crayfish
- o Clams
- o Oysters
- o Scallops

2. **Carbohydrates** - Although the Paleo Diet is practically a low-carbohydrate diet, it doesn't mean that you have to avoid carbs altogether. Since our body still needs carbs for energy, you can get a healthy source of carbs from eating vegetables and fruits.

Vegetables

- o Spinach
- o Lettuce
- o Cabbage
- o Kale
- o Cauliflower
- o Broccoli
- o Brussels sprouts
- o Radish
- o Parsnip
- o Artichoke
- o Asparagus
- o Carrots
- o Squash
- o Pumpkin
- o Cucumber
- o Zucchini
- o Beets
- o Turnips
- o Eggplant
- o Tomatoes
- o Celery
- o All types of peppers

Fruits

- o Bananas
- o Apples
- o Oranges
- o Tangerine
- o Berries (blueberries, strawberries, blackberries)
- o Cherries
- o Cantaloupe
- o Honeydew
- o Watermelon
- o Papaya
- o Mango
- o Kiwi
- o Lemon or Lime
- o Avocado
- o Peaches
- o Nectarines
- o Coconut

3. **Fats** - There's a misconception that fats are bad for the health. But I want you to understand that there is a lot of fats, and they can be found in the following foods:

Oil

- o Olive oil
- o Canola oil
- o Avocado oil
- o Walnut oil

o   Coconut

Nuts and Seeds

o   Almonds

o   Cashews

o   Walnuts

o   Macadamia

o   Hazelnuts

o   Brazil Nuts

o   Pumpkin Seeds

o   Sesame Seeds

o   Sunflower Seeds

4. **Herbs and Spices** - listed below are items you can use to flavor your Paleo dishes

- o Basil
- o Oregano
- o Chili powder
- o Cilantro
- o Black Pepper
- o Cumin
- o Curry

Foods to Avoid

To further guide you to your Paleo Transition, here are some food types that you should avoid.

1. **Dairy**
- o Butter
- o Yoghurt
- o Cheese
- o Any type of meat (skim, whole, powdered, low-fat)
- o Ice cream

2. **Beverages**
- o Manufactured fruit juices
- o Soft drinks
- o Energy drinks
- o Coffee

3. **Grains and Legumes**
- o Rice
- o Peanuts
- o Cereals

4. Processed foods- avoid anything "instant."
o Canned goods
o Nuggets
o Instant noodles
o Microwaveable dinners
o Hotdogs
o Sausage

5. **Fast food**

6. **Salt**

7. **Refined Vegetable Oils**

Chapter 4: The Paleo Diet Effect of Anti-Aging

According to medical journals, a large percentage of chronic diseases and biological aging are as a result of diet, lifestyle and exercise factors. Unfortunately, little standard medical education is directed to these areas. Therefore, the best advice concerning the lifestyles, movement and nutrition are turning to Paleo diet. Paleo foods help a dieter to maintain the youthful energy and vigor, as well as slows down the aging process. What's the connection between Paleo diets and anti-aging? Here's how Paleo diets slow down biological aging:

Enhances positive mood

As people age, it is common for their motivation and mood to wane. According to research, low mood can be associated with low testosterone levels, low omega-3 status, low vitamin D, and high insulin and blood sugars. A majority of the Standard American Diets are rich in simple and processed carbs, which are responsible for weight gain, reduced essential omega-3 fats and vitamin D levels in the blood, inflammation, and insulin dysfunction.

The Paleo approach to dieting provides building blocks to a dieter's body to correct any dysfunction and deficiencies, as well as, improving a person's vitality, as they age.

However, cardio and strength training is also important for mood improvement. Exercise coupled with a low-carb diet is the best approach to reducing stress, blood pressure and bolster health.

Lowers All-Cause Mortality

Recent reports by health experts show that a person's quantity of lean muscle is a key marker for aging healthily. According to the American Journal of Clinical Nutrition, mortality, especially in men with over 80 years, is inversely correlated with the lean muscle mass. Aging healthily or tapping into "the fountain of youth" is possible if a person maintains his muscles. Although the anti-aging benefits of lean muscles accrue to everyone, the co-relation is not common in women.

However, to boost and effectively maintain your lean muscles, you need to incorporate the right food type in your menu. Which food type or diet is the best in increasing lean muscles? Well, a Paleo diet is the answer. Some of the foods which increase lean muscles include beef, seafood, poultry, fish and meats of wild game- the Paleo diet staples. These Paleo diet staples are rich and concentrated with branched-chain amino acids and creatine, as well as, essential amino acids which are paramount for lean muscle maintenance and build-up.

It's recommended for male clients to take portions of up to 1.5x the thickness and size of their palm in each meal, whereas females should consume just 1.0x their palm's thickness and size.

Improves brain's cognition

Why should women remain consistent to high protein diets, yet the chances of lean muscles reducing their mortality are minimal? Cognitive health is the best reason. Anti-aging is not all about physical endeavors such as physical activity or exercise; it is more or less, a mental challenge. Maintaining a calm and relaxed mental state is paramount to anti-aging, and this can be done by reducing stress or depression and going Paleo.

As people age, there is a habit they create of relying primarily on tea and toast for meals. A diet of these convenience foods is commonly known as "tea and toast" diet and has the effect of reducing or suppressing the dieter's appetite. It is these foods of high carbs which wreak havoc on the dieter's neurons (brain cells) and causes dementias and cognitive decline.

Hence, this can be combated by adopting and emphasizing on a diet rich in the Paleo diet staples such as abundant vegetables, healthy fats, and lean meats. These staples not only improve brain's cognition but they also ensure that the optimal blood sugar is restored.

Unfortunately, most dieters have a hard time breaking the habit of relying on the "traditional breakfast" of orange juice, cereals, and toast. Other people find it difficult to consume brain-boosting eggs due to the fear and worry of raising their cholesterol levels. However, if this is so, it's advisable to seek consultation with your healthcare practitioner.

Chapter 5: The Paleo Lifestyles

Paleo lifestyles and high-protein diets

Ensuring an optimal intake of proteins doesn't just improve the lean muscles, other key health markers are also improved: cancer risk, blood pressure, inflammation, and blood sugars. The talk that high-protein diets increase heart disease risk may have struck your ears causing you to refrain from such diets. However, Harvard University conducted a study and found out that compared to high-carb diets and low-protein diets, high-protein diets are superior and more effective in reducing blood pressure. High-protein diets also reduce pro-inflammatory triglycerides and increase HDL cholesterol, which is important.

Paleo diets are not limited to protein intake alone. A paleo dieter is also allowed to engage in the abundant consumption of fruits and nutrient-dense vegetables. Ample consumption of alkalinizing fruits and vegetables has the following benefits:

- Provide essential vitamins

- Improve the minerals amounts

- Provide the body with antioxidants

- Protect damage of DNA

- Fight off cancer

- Improved heart health

- Maintains optimal health

As we age, the intake of veggies and proteins (or general appetite) tends to decline. Unfortunately, the intake of the diet of "tea and toast" is not beneficial to the body health since it doesn't contribute to any nutrients to the body. Therefore, it's recommended to adopt a Paleo lifestyle for your overall benefit.

The Paleo lifestyle involves a lot of exercises or physical movement. But it doesn't necessarily have any effect on a person's chronological age. However, a person's biological age mostly depends on his lifestyle choices such as eating and exercising habits. Therefore, an individual who undertakes to live by the paleo lifestyle stands a better chance of reducing and maintaining his biological age. That is, he can stay young and healthy. A Paleo lifestyle ensures that your blood pressure, blood sugar, lipid panels and mood are all healthy and balanced.

Paleo Lifestyle Anti-aging Effects

The attraction to Paleo diets by most people is as a result of its reputation- improving overall health and lose weight. Well, what if there is another benefit of 'living forever young' associated with going Paleo? To be clear, it's a person's biological age that is in question here, but not his chronological age.

Age concept encompasses two different aspects, biological age, and chronological age. Chronological age is the linear fashion of determining the age of a person such as years, months or days. The chronological age of an individual is always moving forward and can never be reversed. On the other hand, a person's biological age is quite flexible. Biological age involves the youthfulness and vibrancy of a person's body. Therefore, the biological age is dependent on your living lifestyle since you can retain a youthful appeal even when your chronological age is way ahead of your outlook appearance.

With the Paleo lifestyle and diet, maintaining a young biological age isn't much of a hassle irrespective of your actual chronological age. A paleo diet regime strongly advocates against physical inactivity and poor eating since these two are the key ingredients to reducing your biological age. If possible, avoid Standard American Lifestyle and Diet as much as you can. Adhering to Paleo diet strictly is the perfect antidote for aging.

Merits of Paleo Lifestyles

Paleo lifestyles deliver on the promise of smoother skin, better sex and sharper mind.

1. Better sex

The worst fear that most men have is that of a poor functioning "manhood" as they age. Sex is believed to be the 'heart' of every intimate relationship. Therefore, most men in their old age seek ways of correcting and improving their erectile dysfunction problems. As a result, the demand for Viagra in the market has increased especially among the old men.

When Viagra pills were first introduced in the market as erectile dysfunction pills (ED), the profits of the pharmaceutical company soared by 38%. Over the years, the sale of Viagra pills has continued to top the sales lists as new businesses join the profitable industry, and this is an apparent indication that a majority of the men depend on these "little blue pills" for better sexual performance. But the question is, why do most men rely on these pills?

The blockage of the blood arteries responsible for supplying the heart with blood might lead to heart attack. Erectile dysfunction (ED) also follows the same order; interference of the blood supply to the penis due to arteries brokerages. Therefore, ED doesn't mean that you lack an erection; it's the overall health that is deficient.

However, ED might also be caused by prostate disease based complications, emotional, psychological, or physical issues, or pelvis and spine injuries. But in America, research shows that a majority of the death cases reported in the United States are caused by heart disease (Heart disease has claimed approximately 500, 000 lives annually). Therefore, it's clear that poor health is the reason for most health complications.

Unfortunately, poor health-related sexual problems don't exclusively affect males only. Nearly 43% of the female population have experienced a few sexual difficulties. The statistics are slightly higher compared to that of men. The common challenges including orgasm failure, painful intercourse, insufficient vaginal lubrication or sexual arousal failures. Sexual dysfunction is mostly common in women who have metabolic syndrome.

However, Paleo diets and lifestyles have a strong influence in reversing or preventing the cardiovascular disease incidences. The Paleo lifestyle recommends that you embrace quality sleep, consistent exercising and reduce stress. Lack of these three factors proves to be detrimental to a person's cardiovascular health. Therefore, when these Paleo lifestyles are addressed, your sexual health stands a chance to improve without necessarily having to consume any Viagra pills.

2. Sharper Mind

Have you ever misplaced your credit card, forgotten your password, or struggled to remember your lecturer's name? Does this mental lapse occur to you often? If yes, do you want to know why these things happen to you!

Similar to our skin, we have a tendency of expecting mental lapse or deterioration of our memory faculties with time or as we age. We believe that our hands are tied in respect to ensuring our cognitive or brain function remains unaffected even as we age. However, that's not true.

According to an experiment carried out by UCLA's David Geffen School of Medicine researchers, when two rats were placed to navigate a maze, there were two outcomes. The rat that took the water that contained fructose had a significantly worse performance compared to the rat whose water was spiked with docosahexaenoic acid (DHA). Similar to the rats, lack of DHA also affects the human brain. Studies show that low DHA in humans is correlated with improved incidents of Alzheimer's disease and dementia.

One of the following SAD diet standards is low DHA levels. Diets rich in DHA (such as Paleo) are beneficial to the body since the only body synthesis limited quantities. That is why DHA, as a fatty acid, is referred to as "essential". The best dietary sources of this "brain food" are fish, for example, mackerel and salmon. Therefore, you should consider eating more quantity of fish and improve your farm-raised seafood prevalence for your brain health.

Unfortunately, wild-caught seafood contains an amount of heavy metals such as mercury similar to other large predatory fish. Therefore, consuming more of this regular seafood may present an undesirable outcome. However, the convenience of Paleo diets is that they provide alternative sources which are still Paleo-friendly options rich in DHA. They include pastured eggs, small fish such as anchovies and grass-fed beef.

Going beyond diet, physical activity also buffers the brain against the aging effects. The brain's endogenous pharmacology can be influenced by the promising intervention of physical activity to improve emotional and cognitive function during old age. In simpler words, your brain stays young when you indulge in a constructive physical activity.

3. Smoother Skin

In the course of time, we often expect to see a reflection of our image in the mirror being roughened, wrinkled and saggy. As a result, we sit down and watch the vitality and vibrancy of our youth slip helplessly away.

For the entrepreneurs, this seemingly inevitable decline has presented a financial opportunity which they can't help but notice and this has seen the flocking of stores with creams, potions, and pills which promise to fight the aging effects which appear on the skin.

Some people even find the superficial solutions as being ineffective and not enough. Thus, they end up paying the nearby plastic surgeon a visit, intending to find help in tucking and nipping the epidermis which is offensive back in line. The good news is that you need not visit any medical expert since the aging problem can be prevented or solved by proper dieting.

According to a recent survey, an average person takes approximately 22 tsp of sugar on a daily basis; high fructose and corn syrup snacks and sweetened soft drinks encompassing the vast majority. Although most people are aware of the adverse effects such as heart disease and diabetes which accrue from this practice, only a few individuals take caution.

Sugar has a detrimental effect on the body. Glycation is one of the effects of the highly reactive nature of sugar, whereby sugar molecules attach themselves to protein collagen anytime the two come into contact. Glycation negatively affects the functions of protein collagen in the body: Collagen is the structural component of most connective tissues such as the skin.

Once the protein collagen bonds with sugar, it becomes fragile and weak and forms compounds referred to as "Advanced Glycation End Products (AGEs)". As a result, the skin ends up sagging due to lack of collagen scaffolding. According to scientists from Netherlands, the quantified effect of glycation is that it increases an individual's perceived age by close to five months with every sugar increase of 1 mm per blood liter.

Fortunately, paleo diets have limited refined carbohydrates and processed sugars that maintain the blood sugar. Therefore, the formation of AGEs in excess is minimized, and the aging process decelerated.

Summary:

Paleo diet and lifestyle is the perfect "Anti-Aging Protocol" to follow. With Paleo lifestyle, the complicated incessant forward time march is significantly slowed down.

Eat a wide range of cooked vegetables, eggs, seeds and nuts, fresh fruits, meats, and seafood, every day. Drink more water but less alcohol. Avoid legumes, processed sea oils, and foods and grains with gluten. Play enough, run fast and lift weights. Keep a distance from your computer and watching TV, during sleep-time. Cultivate healthy hobbies.

Chapter 6: Your 30-Day Challenge Guaranteed to Give Amazing Results

Are you ready for the challenge? Come on, let's do this!

Day 1 Paleo Challenge

Wake up: Drink water right away. Recommended is 8oz.

Morning workout: Raise your calf with your feet turned out, feet straight and feet turned in. Do this 10 times each.

Breakfast: Coco-Paleo Pancakes and 8oz of water

Yes, you can still have pancakes with the Paleo Diet by using coconut flour on your mixture.

Ingredients:

3tbps. Coconut flour

¼ tsp. baking soda

3 medium-sized eggs

1 tbsp. coconut oil

3 tbsp. coconut milk

2 tbsp. apple sauce (unsweetened)

½ tsp. apple cider vinegar

Procedures:

1. In a bowl, mix the coconut flour and eggs until they are smooth. Add the applesauce, coconut oil, milk, baking soda, vinegar and a small amount of honey.

2. Heat a skillet over medium fire and drizzle hot coconut oil. When the pan is hot, add a small amount of the mixture. Cook the pancakes, until they turn golden brown.

3. Serve with blueberries or strawberries on top and drizzle with honey.

Drink 16oz of water by lunch time.

Lunch: Chicken and Avocado Salad Delight

Ingredients:

2 boneless and skinless chicken breasts (cooked and cut into cubes)

1 large avocado (mashed)

2 tbsp. walnuts (chopped)

2 tbsp. fresh cilantro

1 freshly squeezed lime

Salt to taste

Procedures:

1. In a big bowl, combine the cubed chicken and mashed avocado.

2. Throw in the walnuts, finely chopped cilantro, lime juice, and add a pinch of salt to taste.

3. Combine ingredients thoroughly and serve.

Drink another 8oz of water after lunch.

Snack: Homemade Apple Chips

Get a quick sweet fix with these homemade apple chips.

Ingredients:

2 pcs. Honeycrisp apple

1 tsp. cinnamon powder

1 tsp. raw honey

Procedures:

1. Preheat oven to 250°F.

2. Cut the apples in half and remove the seeds. Take a mandolin and slice the apples thinly.

3. Take a baking sheet and lay over with parchment paper.Take the apple slices and lay them separately. Sprinkle the cinnamon powder over the apple slices.

4. Place in the oven and cook or an hour. Flip the apples and cook for another 1 hour. Take out the oven and drizzle with honey.

Consume after cooling or store in an airtight container.

Dinner: Baked Salmon Dinner

This is a simple yet tasty baked salmon recipe.

Ingredients:

1 pc. Wild-caught salmon (32 oz.)

1 lemon (sliced thinly)

1 tbsp. capers

1 tbsp. thyme

Olive oil

Salt and pepper to taste

Procedures:

1. Pre-heat oven to 400°F

2. Prepare a baking sheet and top it with parchment paper. Place the salmon (skin side first) on the sheet and season with salt and pepper.

3. Top the salmon with capers, lemon and fresh thyme and bake in the oven for 25 minutes.

4. Best served, when hot.

Exercise of the day: The Pike

Lie face up with your legs straight, arms at your sides, palms facing down. Raise your legs and torso 45 degrees off the floor. (Your body should look like a "V".) Reach your hands alongside your legs as high as you can without rounding your back.

Start with one set of 8-12 rep. Once you can consistently get 15 reps, add another set.

Bedtime: Drink 16oz of water before you go to bed

Day 2 Paleo Challenge

Wake up: Drink water right away. Recommended is 8oz.

Morning workout: Do 10 push-ups to get your blood flowing

Breakfast: 8oz of water and Heavenly Ham n' Eggs

A simple two-ingredient recipe you'll want to eat, every morning!

Ingredients:

4 slices of ham

2 eggs

(spices for flavor)

Procedures:

1. Preheat your oven to 400 °F

2. Prepare a muffin pan by greasing it with coconut oil.

3. Place two pieces of ham on top of each other in one muffin cup. Repeat with the next muffin cup.

4. Crack the egg on top of the ham

   (Optional: add scallions, basil, etc. on your egg for more flavor)

5. Bake for 15 minutes and serve.

Drink 16oz of water by lunch time.

Lunch: Veggie-bun Sandwich

Ingredients:

1 pc. red bell pepper

2 slices turkey ham

½ avocado (cut into strips)

1 pc. seaweed strips

Procedures:

1. Take the bell pepper and slice it in half and remove the seeds.
2. Take one piece of bell pepper and top it with the ham, seaweed, and avocado.
3. Top with the other half of the bell pepper and stick a toothpick in the center. Enjoy.

Drink another 8oz of water after lunch.

Snack: Celery with 2 tablespoons of sunflower butter or baby carrots and few raisins.

Dinner: Low-carb Paleo Patties and 8oz of water

Ingredients

16 oz. ground lean turkey

1 tsp. Paprika

½ tsp. coriander

1 tsp. powdered onion

a pinch of cayenne pepper

a pinch of salt

a pinch of ground pepper

2 pcs. green onions (chopped)

1 pc. tomato (sliced)

2 cups arugula

1 pc. avocado (sliced)

Procedures:

1. In a bowl, place the ground turkey and add the onion powder, salt, pepper, paprika, cayenne pepper, and green onions and combine everything.

2. Use your hands to form into burger patties.

3. Heat the grill and cook the burgers for 5 minutes, per side.

4. Place the cooked patties over the arugula, tomatoes, and avocado. Serve.

Exercise of the day: Tree-pose Yoga

This pose will have your abdominals working overtime to help you stay grounded on one leg.

Shift your weight onto your left foot. Draw your right knee into your chest, grab your ankle, and press the bottom of your right foot onto your left thigh. If you feel wobbly, keep your hand on your ankle while it is pressed into your thigh. If you're finding your balance easily, press your palms together in front of your chest. Brace your abdominals in tight to your spine, making sure you can still breathe easily. Find a focal point and focus your gaze while you hold the pose for ten long, deep breaths. Repeat on the other leg.

Bedtime: Drink 8oz of water before you go to bed

Day 3 Paleo Challenge

Wake up: Drink water right away. Recommended is 8oz.

Morning workout: Raise your calf with your feet turned out, feet straight and feet turned in. Do this 10 times each.

Breakfast: Kale Breakfast Muffin and 8oz of water

Ingredients:

½ cup kale (finely chopped)

1/8 cup onion chives (finely chopped)

¼ cup almond milk

3 eggs

4 slices of smoked turkey

Pepper to taste

Procedures:

1. Preheat oven at 350 °F

2. In a mixing bowl, whisk together the eggs, kale, chives, almond milk and sprinkle with pepper to taste

3. Take a muffin pan and grease it with coconut oil. Fill the muffin cups with two slices of smoked turkey each and fill 2/3 of it with the kale mixture.

4. Bake for 30 minutes. Let it cool and serve.

Drink 16oz of water by lunch time.

Lunch: Cucumber Sandwich

Ingredients:

1 pc.cucumber

3 slices turkey breast slices (low sodium)

Dijon mustard

Garlic and herb spreadable

Procedures:

1. Take the cucumber and cut in half. Remove the seeds.

2. Spread the garlic and herb on cucumber.

3. Add lay the turkey slices on top and drizzle with Dijon mustard.

4. Sandwich with the other half of the cucumber. Enjoy.

Drink another 8oz of water after lunch.

Snack: Berry-coconut Shake

Ingredients:

8 pcs. frozen strawberries

1 cup coconut milk

1 tsp. honey

1 tsp. almond butter

2 pcs. fresh strawberries

Coconut shavings

Procedures:

1. Blend the strawberries, coconut milk, honey and almond butter.

2. Top with sliced fresh strawberries and coconut shavings.

Dinner: Slow-cooked Chicken Zing and 8oz of water

A zesty take on your favorite chicken!

Ingredients:

48 oz. chicken legs (drumsticks)

1/3 cup fresh orange juice

2 tsp. orange zest

¼ cup raw honey

3 cloves garlic (minced)

1 tbsp. grated ginger

1 tbsp. coconut aminos

½ tbsp. balsamic vinegar

1 tsp. tomato paste

1 tbsp. sesame seeds

(optional) ½ tbsp. Sriracha sauce

green onions (chopped)

sesame seeds

Procedures:

1. Whisk all the ingredients in a bowl (except chicken).
2. Season the chicken with salt and pepper and place in a slow cooker and pour the sauce. Place in a slow cooker and cook over low heat for 4 hours.
3. Place the chicken on a plate and put the sauce in a small pan. Simmer the sauce for 15 minutes. Pour the sauce over the chicken and garnish with green onions and sesame seeds.

Exercise of the day: Side Plank

Lie on your left side with your elbow directly beneath your shoulder and legs stacked. Place your right hand on your left shoulder or your right hip.

Brace your abs and lift your hips off the floor until you're balancing on your forearm and feet so that your body forms a diagonal line. Hold for 30 to 45 seconds. If you can't hold that long, stay up as long as you can and then repeat until you've held for 30 seconds total. Switch sides and repeat.

This abs exercise is more challenging than a traditional plank because you're supporting your entire body weight on two points of contact instead of four. As a result, you must work your core harder to stay stabilized.

Bedtime: Drink 8oz of water before you go to bed

Day 4 Paleo Challenge

Wake up: Drink water right away. Recommended is 8oz.

Morning workout: Do 10 push-ups to get your blood flowing

Breakfast: 8oz of water and Easy-o-whip Gluten-Free Banana Pancakes

Enjoy this delicious breakfast in just three easy steps!

Ingredients:

¼ teaspoon baking powder

4 eggs

2 large bananas (chopped)

Procedures:

1. Place the ingredients in a bowl and mix with an immersion blender.

2. Heat a non-stick pan over medium-high heat.

3. Ladle the batter and place in the pan one at a time. Cook until the pancake bubbles, then flip and cook for another 30 seconds. Serve.

Drink 16oz of water by lunch time.

Lunch: Prosciutto Wrapped Chicken

A delicious and protein rich meal.

Ingredients:

3 pcs. chicken legs

1 tbsp. coconut oil

1 small shallot (chopped)

2 garlic cloves (minced)

2 cups spinach (frozen, roughly chopped)

1/3 cup olives (chopped)

3 slices prosciutto

1 tbsp. olive oil

salt and pepper to taste

Procedures:

1. Preheat oven at 325°F
2. Heat the pan over medium fire and drizzle with coconut oil.
3. Saute the garlic and shallots for 2 minutes.
4. Toss in the spinach and olives and cook for 5 minutes.
5. Remove from the heat and set in a bowl.
6. Top the mixture on the chicken thigh and wrap each leg with a slice of prosciutto.
7. Take a ceramic baking dish and drizzle with olive oil. Place the chicken on the dish and bake in the oven for an hour, or until the internal temperature reached 155°F.

Drink another 8oz of water after lunch.

Snack: Green Paleo Smoothie

This healthy and refreshing drink will not only quench your thirst but will also satisfy your cravings for sweets.

Ingredients:

1 pc. mango (diced)

2 cups kale (stems removed)

½ lime (juiced)

1 pc. kiwi (diced)

1 cup coconut milk

water

Procedures:

1. Blend all the ingredients together, adding water to achieve your preferred consistency.

Dinner: Beef Skewers and 8oz of water

Start the grill and cook these beef kebabs for dinner!

Ingredients:

32 oz. sirloin beef (cut into 2" cubes)

1 pc. zucchini (cut into 1" cubes)

1 onion (cut into 1"squares)

1 red or green bell pepper (cut into 1" squares)

Marinade

5 garlic cloves

1 small onion (chopped)

¼ cup squeezed orange juice

1 tsp. orange zest

1 tbsp. rosemary (chopped)

¼ cup olive oil

2 tbsp. organic tomato paste

sea salt and pepper to taste

Procedures:

1. Combine all the marinade recipes in a food processor until you reach a smooth paste. Set aside ¼ cup of the marinade for the veggies.

2. In a bowl, place beef and pour over the marinade. Toss the beef to make sure that it is well-coated with the marinade. Refrigerate it overnight.

3. When you're ready to cook, remove the beef in the fridge 30 minutes before grilling, to allow it to thaw.

4. Take the ¼ cup marinade and toss it with the vegetables in a bowl.

5. Thread the beef cubes and vegetables alternately using bamboo or metal skewers.

6. Bring the grill over medium heat and cook the kebabs, turning each side after four minutes. The whole kebab will cook in about 12 minutes or until it is well-cooked.

Exercise of the day: Walkout from Pushup Position

Start in pushup position with hands two inches wider than your shoulders.

Walk hands out as far as possible, then walk back. Do 10-12 reps.

Bedtime: Drink 8oz of water before you go to bed

Day 5 Paleo Challenge

Wake up: Drink water right away. Recommended is 8oz.

Morning workout: Raise your calf with your feet turned out, feet straight and feet turned in. Do this 10 times each.

Breakfast: 8oz of water and Paleo-friendly Banana Loaf

Who says you can't eat bread when you go Paleo? Try this Paleo-friendly recipe for a breakfast loaf!

Ingredients:

4 large bananas (mashed)

4 tbsp. Coconut oil (or grass-fed butter)

4 eggs

½ cup almond flour (you can also use coconut flour as a substitute)

1 tsp. baking soda

1 tsp. gluten-free baking powder

1 tsp. cinnamon powder

½ cup almond butter

1 tsp. vanilla extract

a pinch of sea salt

Procedures:

1. Preheat oven at 350°F

2. In a bowl, mix the bananas, eggs, and coconut oil and blend well using a hand mixer.

3. Once all the ingredients are well-blended, add the almond flour, cinnamon, baking powder, baking soda, vanilla and sea salt. Mix well.

4. Grease a loaf pan and pour the batter. Cook in the oven for an hour, until its color turns into golden brown.

5. Flip the cooked loaf on a cooling rack. Slice and serve.

Drink 16oz of water by lunch time.

Lunch: Perfect Paleo Meatloaf

This is a perfect Paleo-friendly meatloaf you can cook, especially on Sunday dinners.

Ingredients:

32 oz. lean, organic pork (ground)

10 oz. thawed frozen spinach (squeeze excess water)

1 onion (diced)

6 oz. mushrooms (diced)

2 pcs. carrots (diced)

4 eggs (beaten)

2 tsp. olive oil

2 tsp. sea salt

2 tsp. freshly ground pepper

2 tsp. onion powder

1 tsp. thyme

1 tsp. garlic powder

1/3 cup coconut flour

¼ tsp. grated nutmeg

Procedures:

1. Preheat oven at 375°F

2. Place a pan on medium fire and drizzle with olive oil. Saute the onions and mushrooms, until the onions are caramelized. Remove from the heat and let it cool.

3. In a large bowl, combine the meat, chopped spinach, cooked onions and mushrooms, eggs, spices and coconut flour. Mix well with your hands, making sure to break up the meat.

4. Grease a loaf pan and fill with the meat mixture.

5. Cook in the oven for about 25 minutes, or until the internal temperature reaches 160°F.

6. After cooking, remove from the oven and let it cool before serving.

Drink another 8oz of water after lunch.

Snack: Homemade Apple Chips (repeat day one snack)

Get a quick sweet fix with these homemade apple chips.

Ingredients:

2 pcs. Honeycrisp apple

1 tsp. cinnamon powder

1 tsp. raw honey

Procedures:

1. Preheat oven to 250°F.

2. Cut the apples in half and remove the seeds. Take a mandolin and slice the apples thinly.

3. Take a baking sheet and lay over with the parchment paper.Take the apple slices and lay them separately. Sprinkle the cinnamon powder over the apple slices.

4. Place in the oven and cook or an hour. Flip the apples and cook for another 1 hour. Take out the oven and drizzle with honey.

Consume after cooling or store in an airtight container.

Dinner: Grilled Pork Chops with Pear Relish and 8oz of water

This meaty, fruity combo is a recipe you'll enjoy eating!

Ingredients:

2 pcs. pork chops

¼ cup mustard

1 cup pear (pitted and diced)

1 small shallot (diced)

1/8 cup fresh basil (finely chopped)

1 ½ tbsp. apple cider vinegar

1/8 cup olive oil

Procedures:

1. Marinate pork chops in a salt and pepper rub for 30 mins.
2. In a mixing bowl, combine the mustard, pear, diced shallot, basil, vinegar, olive oil and set aside.
3. When marinated, place the chops on a preheated grill and cook for six minutes each side.
4. Serve pork chops with peach relish on top.

Exercise of the day: The Pike

Lie face up with your legs straight, arms at your sides, palms facing down. Raise your legs and torso 45 degrees off the floor. (Your body should look like a "V".) Reach your hands alongside your legs as high as you can without rounding your back.

Start with one set of 8-12 rep. Once you can consistently get 15 reps, add another set.

Bedtime: Drink 8oz of water before you go to bed

Day 6 Paleo Challenge

Wake up: Drink water right away. Recommended is 8oz.

Morning workout: Do 10 push-ups to get your blood flowing

Breakfast: 8oz of water and Homemade Corned Beef

Have corned beef and radishes (instead of potatoes) with this recipe!

Ingredients:

2 cups corned beef (cooked and chopped)

3 cups radishes (cut into quarters)

1 small onion (chopped)

2 garlic cloves (minced)

½ cup beef broth

salt and pepper to taste

Procedures:

1. Heat a pan over medium-high heat and drizzle with oil.

2. Saute the onions for 4 minutes and then add radishes. Cook for another 5 minutes.

3. Add the garlic and sauté for another minute.

4. Pour in the broth and then cover loosely. Let it simmer for five minutes or until the radishes are tender.

5. Add the corned beef and stir well.

6. Season with a dash of salt and pepper.

Drink 16oz of water by lunch time.

Lunch: Chicken Salad

Servings: 2

Ingredients:

2 chicken breasts, skinned and deboned

1 avocado

2 tbsp cilantro

2 tbsp avocado

3 tbsp lime juice

1 tbsp coconut oil

sea salt

Procedures:

1. Heat pan to high and put oil, cook chicken. When cooked, cut chicken into small cubes
2. Place chicken in salad bowl and add rest of the ingredients
3. Add salt to taste
4. Serve

Drink another 8oz of water after lunch.

Snack: Apple with sunflower butter

Dinner: Seared Steak and 8oz of water

Servings: 2

Ingredients:

2 rib eye steaks

1 tbsp of rosemary

1 tbsp butter

1/4 tsp garlic powder

1/4 tsp onion powder

1/4 tsp paprika

1 tbsp coconut oil

5 cloves garlic

sea salt and black pepper

Procedures:

1. Create the steak rub by combining the garlic, onion and paprika powder with salt. Set aside when combined.
2. Heat pan on high for 2 minutes
3. Rub the oil into the steaks
4. Take steak rub and sprinkle on the steak
5. Put steak on pan and cook for 3 minutes on each side
6. Remove steak and put on plate
7. Lower the heat of pan and put rosemary, garlic and butter
8. Cook for 2 minutes, stir occasionally
9. Drip the butter mixture on the steaks
10. Serve

Exercise of the day: Warrior III

This yoga move can tone your legs, and core too.

Stand with the feet together, and lift up the left leg with a pointed toe, putting your body weight on the standing, right foot. Continue to lift your leg and drop the head and torso so they form a straight horizontal line from head to toe with the arms at your sides. Engage your core and make sure the left thigh, hip, and toes are aligned. Remain facing down and keep your back as straight as possible. Ensure your right knee doesn't lock and centers the weight on the middle of the foot. Hold for 5 breaths and then slowly return to standing.

Switch legs and repeat.

Bedtime: Drink 8oz of water before you go to bed

Day 7 Paleo Challenge

Wake up: Drink water right away. Recommended is 8oz.

Morning workout: Raise your calf with your feet turned out, feet straight and feet turned in. Do this 10 times each.

Breakfast: 8oz of water and Banana-berry Toast

Have this sweet and filling breakfast to jumpstart your day!

Ingredients:

1 loaf Paleo banana bread (refer to recipe 5)

1 cup blueberries (frozen)

1 cup coconut milk

5 eggs

¼ cup raw honey

1 tsp. vanilla extract

1 tsp. ground cinnamon

Procedures:

1. Preheat oven at 350°F
2. Cut the loaf into cubes and place in a baking dish (8x8") with the blueberries
3. In a mixing bowl, blend the coconut milk,honey, cinnamon, vanilla, and eggs.
4. Pour the mixture on the bread and berries and bake for 45 minutes.
5. When cooked, remove from the oven and allow to cool for 15 minutes. Serve.

Drink 16oz of water by lunch time

Lunch: Salmon Glaze

Servings: 2

Ingredients:

12 oz. salmon fillets

2 tbsp honey

1 tbsp coconut oil

2 tbsp coconut aminos

1 tbsp apple cider vinegar

1 tbsp grated ginger

1 tsp sesame seeds

1/2 tsp lime juice

1 tbsp chopped cilantro

Procedures:

1. Heat oven to 400 degrees
2. In a bowl, combine aminos, vinegar, honey and lime juice. Set aside.
3. Heat pan to high and put coconut oil
4. Sear salmon with the skin side of the fillet up until brown
5. When brown, flip salmon and drizzle honey glaze
6. Bake for 5 minutes
7. Remove and drizzle again with honey
8. Add garnishes, cilantro and seeds
9. Serve

Drink another 8oz of water after lunch.

Snack: Energy Bars

Servings: 5 bars

Ingredients:

•1 medium, banana (very ripe works best)

•1/4 cup nuts (I used salted cashews)

•1/3 cup dried fruit (I used cherries)

•1/4 cup seeds (I used sunflower seeds, or sub for more nuts)

•1/4 cup vanilla protein powder (try with another flavor and let me know how it is)

•2 tbsp arrowroot starch (or other starch)

•1/2 cup almond flour (thought I should add parenthesis here too)

Procedures:

1. In a bowl, mash the banana well with a fork or other handy utensil. It doesn't have to be perfect.

2. Add almond flour and arrowroot starch and mix well.

3. Add in your mix-ins and stir well.

4. Grease a small pan (I used a meatloaf pan and it was perfect) with your favorite oil and pour mixture in, pressing down where needed to evenly distribute throughout.

5. Bake on around 275 for 30-40 minutes, or until the edges start to brown.

6. Take out the loaf, and cut into cute bars or squares.

Power up as needed! And store in the fridge after a day.

Dinner: Thai Chicken and 8oz of water

Servings: 4

Ingredients:

1 lb. chicken breasts, deboned and skinned

12 lettuce leaves

3 onions, sliced

1 carrot, shredded

1 broccoli, cut into florets

¼ cup cilantro

2 tbsp coconut aminos

2 tbsp lime juice

Water

Procedures:

1. Cook chicken and cut into small cubes
2. Take lettuce and spread on flat surface
3. Add chicken, carrots, cilantro and onions
4. Drizzle with aminos and lime juice
5. Serve

Exercise of the day: 20 minute Killer Core Workout

As this is a longer workout, it is recommended that you follow the workout in the video below. Push yourself hard tonight as this is the last workout of the week! Drink plenty of water throughout the exercise.

Workout video → https://www.youtube.com/watch?v=KUjFh4J1dnc

Bedtime: Drink 8oz of water before you go to bed

Day 8 Paleo Challenge

Wake up: Drink water right away. Recommended is 8oz.

Morning workout: Do 10 push-ups to get your blood flowing

Breakfast: 8oz of water and Egg Muffin

Servings: 2

Ingredients:

1 cup lean meat, cooked and shredded

9 eggs

1 tsp paprika

3 tbsp coconut milk

1/2 cup tomatoes

1 onion, minced

1 tbsp coconut oil

sea salt and black pepper

Procedures:

1. Heat oven to 350 degrees
2. Heat pan on medium and put oil
3. Sauté onions for 5 minutes
4. Turn off heat and add meat. Set aside
5. Use a bowl and put together milk, eggs, salt and pepper. Set aside
6. Put liners on muffin tin and add egg mixture
7. Add pinch paprika on top of each muffin
8. Put in oven and cook for 30 minutes
9. Serve

Drink 16oz of water by lunch time.

Lunch: Beef & Noodles

Servings: 3

Ingredients:

1/4 lb. flank steak, cubed

1/2 pack squash noodles

1 egg scrambled and sliced into thin pieces

1/2 tbsp coconut oil

2 tbsp coconut aminos

1/4 cup bone broth

1 cup spinach

1/2 cup carrots, shredded

1/4 onion, sliced

2 cloves garlic, minced

1 stalk of green onion

1/2 tbsp sesame oil

1/2 tbsp sesame seeds

1/2 tsp fish sauce

1/2 pack mushrooms

Procedures:

1. Submerge spinach in boiling water and drain as soon as possible, completely dry by patting with paper towel. Mix sesame oil. Set aside and let cool.
2. Sauté garlic and onion in coconut oil add steak and cook until brown
3. Put in aminos, broth, carrots, mushrooms, eggs and fish sauce
4. Allow broth to simmer
5. Add noodles and stir occasionally
6. Cover and allow noodles to absorb the broth
7. Remove from heat and add the onions, spinach and seeds
8. Serve

Drink another 8oz of water after lunch.

Snack: Celery with 2 tablespoons of sunflower butter or baby carrots and few raisins.

Dinner: Mackerel with Cabbage and 8oz of water

Servings: 5

Ingredients:

4 mackerel fillets

1 egg

3 tbsp olive oil

1/2 cup almond flour

1/4 tsp mustard powder

sea salt and black pepper

1 head cabbage

6 cloves garlic

2 cups broccoli florets

1 cup chicken broth

1 tbsp coconut oil

Procedures:
1. For the fish
2. Heat oven to 350 degrees
3. Whisk egg and set aside
4. Use a plate and put together flour, mustard, salt and pepper
5. Dip mackerel in egg and then in flour mixture
6. Heat skillet to medium, put oil and fry for 2 minutes
7. Put in oven for 10 minutes
8. For the cabbage
9. Heat skillet to medium and put oil
10. Sauté garlic until fragrant and add cabbage, stir again

11. Add florets and cook for 1 minute
12. Pour broth and bring to a simmer
13. Take out fish from oven and put in plate
14. Put cabbage on small bowl and serve as a side

Exercise of the day: The Pike

Lie face up with your legs straight, arms at your sides, palms facing down. Raise your legs and torso 45 degrees off the floor. (Your body should look like a "V".) Reach your hands alongside your legs as high as you can without rounding your back.

Start with one set of 8-12 rep. Once you can consistently get 15 reps, add another set.

Bedtime: Drink 8oz of water before you go to bed

Day 9 Paleo Challenge

Wake up: Drink water right away. Recommended is 8oz.

Morning workout: Raise your calf with your feet turned out, feet straight and feet turned in. Do this 10 times each.

Breakfast: 8oz of water and Paleo Breakfast

Servings: 6

Ingredients:

3/4 lb. steak, slice into small pieces

4 eggs

2 sweet potatoes, chop into cubes

1 red bell pepper, chopped

1 green bell pepper, chopped

1 tomato, diced

2 tbsp. coconut oil

sea salt and black pepper to taste

Procedures:

1. Pre-heat oven to 350 degrees
2. Put oil in skillet and set to high
3. Put steak, cook until brown and then set aside
4. Sauté peppers and onions for 5 minutes
5. Add potatoes and cook for 10 minutes
6. Add steak and combine ingredients together
7. Use a spoon and dig small scoops in the potato mixture
8. Crack the eggs into the scoops
9. Put tomatoes on top of the eggs
10. Add salt and pepper to taste
11. Bake for 10 minutes

Drink 16oz of water by lunch time.

Lunch: Spaghetti & Sausage

Servings: 4

Ingredients:

4 Italian sausages

1 squash

8 oz. tomato sauce, organic

2 tbsp olive oil

2 tsp oregano

2 tsp basil

2 tsp thyme

6 clove garlic

Procedures:

1. Put oil, herbs, garlic and sauce on slow cooker and set to high
2. Halve the squash and remove the seeds
3. Add squash on cooker and put on slow cooker
4. Cut sausages into small pieces and add to cooker. Leave for 3 hours
5. Take squash from cooker and scrape flesh using fork, this creates the pasta
6. Put pasta on plate and top with the sauce
7. Serve

Drink another 8oz of water after lunch.

Snack: Berry-coconut Shake

Ingredients:

8 pcs. frozen strawberries

1 cup coconut milk

1 tsp. honey

1 tsp. almond butter

2 pcs. fresh strawberries

Coconut shavings

Procedures:

1. Blend the strawberries, coconut milk, honey and almond butter.
2. Top with sliced fresh strawberries and coconut shavings.

Dinner: Snapper

Servings: 4

Ingredients:

1 lb. red snapper fillet

1 bell pepper , chopped

¼ cup cilantro

1 onion, cut into thin slices

1 tomato, chopped

1 tbsp lemon juice

1 tbsp lime juice

1 tsp chili powder

Black pepper

Procedures:

1. Heat oven to 350 degrees

2. Put fish on baking dish
3. Drizzle lime and lemon juice and sprinkle chili powder
4. Leave for 10 minutes, turn every few minutes
5. Chop onions, peppers and tomato and sprinkle of top of fish
6. Cover and put in oven for 30 minutes
7. Allow 5 minutes outside the oven
8. Garnish with cilantro
9. Serve

Exercise of the day: Single Leg Lift and Row

This move works more than just the legs; it targets the back, arms, and core in addition to the butt and hamstrings.

Begin standing with your left foot in front of the right foot. Hold a 5- to 8-pound dumbbell in the right hand and keep both arms at your sides. Leaning forward, raise the right foot off the ground and bring it straight up to hip level. At the same time, bring the weight toward the ground and then raise it up to hip-level.

Do 12-15 reps on the right side before switching arms and legs to repeat on the left side.

Bedtime: Drink 8oz of water before you go to bed

Day 10 Paleo Challenge

Wake up: Drink water right away. Recommended is 8oz.

Morning workout: Do 10 push-ups to get your blood flowing

Breakfast: 8oz of water and Old Fashioned Pancakes

Servings: 2

Ingredients:

3 eggs

4 bananas

1/4 cup almond butter

1 tbsp coconut oil

Procedures:

1. Put banana and eggs in a bowl and mash together until smooth
2. Add butter, mix again until creamy
3. Put pan on heat and heat oil
4. Pour batter and cook until golden brown

Drink 16oz of water by lunch time.

Lunch: Turkey Sandwich

Servings: 2

Ingredients:

6 slices of turkey breast, cooked

1 cucumber

1 tbsp Dijon mustard

1 tsp garlic powder

1 tsp red pepper flakes

2 tbsp low-fat mayonnaise

Procedures:

1. Remove cucumber seeds and cut into small pieces and set aside
2. Make the spread by putting together garlic powder, pepper flakes and mayonnaise. Spread on the cucumber slices.
3. Put turkey slices and spread mustard on top
4. Serve

Drink another 8oz of water after lunch.

Snack: Green Paleo Smoothie

This healthy and refreshing drink will not only quench your thirst but will also satisfy your cravings for sweets.

Ingredients:

1 pc. mango (diced)

2 cups kale (stems removed)

½ lime (juiced)

1 pc. kiwi (diced)

1 cup coconut milk

water

Procedures:

1. Blend all the ingredients together, adding water to achieve your preferred consistency.

Dinner: Shrimp & Cauliflower

Servings: 2

Ingredients:

1/2 lb shrimp, remove vein and shell

1 head cauliflower

1/2 cup peas

1/2 cup carrots, chopped into thin slices

1 yellow squash, chopped

1 bell pepper, chopped

1/4 tsp red pepper flakes

1 tbsp minced ginger

1 tsp coconut oil

sea salt and black pepper

Procedures:

1. Grate cauliflower into a rice-like consistency
2. Put skillet on medium heat, put oil. Sauté onion and garlic
3. Add cauliflower, salt and pepper. Cook for 5 minutes and set aside
4. Put oil and add pepper flakes, garlic and ginger and cook for 2 minutes
5. Add carrots, bell pepper, peas and squash and fry until bright in color and set aside
6. Put oil and add shrimp and ginger, fry until shrimp is pink
7. Add vegetables for 2 minutes
8. Add cauliflower rice and stir for 2 minutes
9. Serve

Exercise of the day: 10 minutes routine (repeat 3 times)

1. The long-arm crunch 12 reps

2. Reverse crunch 12 reps

3. Janda sit-up 12 reps

4. The Jacknife 12 reps

5. Extended plank 45 seconds

1. The long-arm crunch

Lie on your back with your knees bent and your arms straightened behind you. Then, keeping your arms straight above your head, perform a traditional crunch. The movement should be slow and controlled.

2. The reverse crunch

Lie on your back and place your hands behind your head, then bring your knees in towards your chest until they're bent to 90 degrees, with feet together or crossed. Contract your abs to curl your hips off the floor, reaching your legs up towards the ceiling, then lower your legs back down to their original position without letting your feet touch the floor. This ensures your abs are continually activated.

3. Janda sit-up

Lie on your back with your knees bent and hands placed behind your head. Then try 'digging' your heels into the floor, contracting your hamstrings, whilst performing an ordinary crunch.

4. The Jacknife

Place a mat on the floor, lie down on your back and extend your arms above your head. Simultaneously lift your arms and legs toward the ceiling, until your fingertips touch your toes, then return to your starting position.

5. The extended plank

Get into a press-up position, placing your hands around 10 inches in front of your shoulders, with the toes of your shoes placed against the floor. Hold this position with your back straight and try to continue to breathe as normal.

Bedtime: Drink 8oz of water before you go to bed

<u>Day 11 Paleo Challenge</u>

Wake up: Drink water right away. Recommended is 8oz.

Morning workout: Do 10 push-ups to get your blood flowing

Breakfast: 8oz of water and Egg Breakfast

Servings: 2

Ingredients:

2 eggs

1 tbsp coconut oil

1 cup spinach, chopped

1 cup broccoli flowers, cooked

1/2 avocado, cut into small chunks

1 /2 cup tomatoes cut into small sizes

sea salt and black pepper

Procedures:

1. Heat pan on low and put coconut oil
2. Cook sunny side eggs
3. Put vegetable ingredients, except avocado, on bowl and toss
4. Put eggs on top of vegetables
5. Add salt and pepper to taste
6. Top with avocado
7. Serve

Drink 16oz of water by lunch time.

Lunch: Spinach and Pancetta Frittatas

Servings: 4 - 6

Ingredients:

6 eggs

1/3 cup coconut milk

3 oz diced pancetta

1/2 cup diced onion

2 cups shredded raw sweet potato

2 cups fresh spinach leaves

salt, pepper, any other favorite seasonings

Procedures:

1. In a mixing bowl, whisk the eggs
2. Add the coconut milk, salt, pepper, any other herbs or seasoning you like. Stir and set aside.
3. Preheat oven to 350° F
4. Brown the pancetta over medium heat on an oven-proof frying pan. When browned, remove pancetta but leave the fat in frying pan
5. Add the onions and shredded sweet potatoes – cook in the pancetta fat for about 3 minutes
6. Add spinach to frying pan and cook until leaves start to wilt
7. Now take your bowl of whisked eggs and pour over the potatoes, onions and spinach in the frying pan
8. Allow to cook for about 2 minutes, then sprinkle the pancetta on top
9. Transfer the pan to the preheated 350° F oven and bake for 20-25 minutes until cooked through
10. Remove from oven and allow it to rest for a minute or two
11. Slice and serve!

Note: You may use fried and chopped bacon strips if pancetta is unavailable

Drink another 8oz of water after lunch.

Snack: Apple with sunflower butter

Dinner: Fish Sticks and 8oz of water

Servings: 12 sticks

Ingredients:

1/2 lb cream dory fillets

2 eggs

1 tbsp coconut oil

2 cups almond flour

sea salt and black pepper

Procedures:

1. Put eggs in bowl and whisk
2. Use bowl and put together flour, salt and pepper
3. Heat skillet to medium and put in oil
4. Cut fillets into thin strips, dip in egg mixture and then in flour
5. Fry for 2 minutes
6. Remove fish sticks and put in paper towel
7. Serve

Exercise of the day: Rock 'n Roll Lotus

Sit with your legs crossed at the ankles. Hold onto the outside of each ankle with your opposite hand, and lift your legs off the floor, balancing on your sitting bones. Pull your abs into your spine and take a deep breath in. As you exhale, begin to round onto your back. Continue rolling until your shoulder blades touch the floor, lifting your hips, still holding onto your ankles. Keeping your abs in tight, rock back up to sitting, finding your balance again on your sitting bones. That's one rep. Repeat 10 times.

Imagine you are using your abs as brakes to help you stop at the top and bottom of the rocking motion.

Bedtime: Drink 8oz of water before you go to bed

Day 12 Paleo Challenge

Wake up: Drink water right away. Recommended is 8oz.

Morning workout: Raise your calf with your feet turned out, feet straight and feet turned in. Do this 10 times each.

Breakfast: 8oz of water and Paleo Blueberry Muffin

Ingredients:

2 1/2 cups almond meal (almond flour)

3 large eggs, fresh

1/2 cups Cooper's pure raw honey

1/2 tsp baking powder

1/2 tsp salt

1 tbsp vanilla extract

1 cup blueberries, fresh

Procedures:

1. Preheat oven to 300°.
2. Line a 6 cup muffin pan with muffin liners.
3. In a large bowl, mix all ingredients together, except blueberries, until full combined. Gently fold in blueberries.
4. Fill each liner 3/4 full with batter.
5. Bake for 30-40 minutes. (Top should be spongy, but firm when pressed.)
6. Cool for 5 minutes and remove from muffin pan.

Drink 16oz of water by lunch time.

Lunch: Vegan Salad

Servings: 2

Ingredients:

2 cups mushrooms

2 cups cucumber, sliced

2 cups spinach, chopped

2 cups lettuce, torn

1/4 cup carrot, sliced

1/4 cup cucumber, sliced

1/4 cup onion, sliced

1 tbsp coconut oil

1 tbsp olive oil

Procedures:

Put skillet on high heat and put coconut oil

Sauté onion, garlic, mushrooms and spinach for 5 minute and set aside

Toss remaining ingredients, except olive oil, in bowl

Take tossed ingredients and sautéed vegetables and put together

Drizzle with olive oil

Serve

Drink another 8oz of water after lunch.

Snack: Celery with 2 tablespoons of sunflower butter or baby carrots and few raisins.

Dinner: Chicken Pesto

Servings: 2

Ingredients:

2 chicken breasts

1/2 cup basil leaves

1/3 cup walnuts, chopped

2 cloves garlic

1 tsp rosemary leaves, dried

2 tbsp EVOO

sea salt and black pepper

Procedures:

1. Heat oven to 375 degrees
2. Put basil, garlic, walnuts and oil in a food process, blend until pasty texture
3. Create a flap on the chicken breast and use heavy object to flatten the breast
4. Stuff pesto paste in breast, reseal with the flap
5. Put salt and pepper to taste and bake for 30 minutes
6. Serve

Exercise of the day: 10 minutes routine (repeat 3 times)

1. The long-arm crunch 12 reps

2. Reverse crunch 12 reps

3. Janda sit-up 12 reps

4. The Jacknife 12 reps

5. Extended plank 45 seconds

1. The long-arm crunch

Lie on your back with your knees bent and your arms straightened behind you. Then, keeping your arms straight above your head, perform a traditional crunch. The movement should be slow and controlled.

2. The reverse crunch

Lie on your back and place your hands behind your head, then bring your knees in towards your chest until they're bent to 90 degrees, with feet together or crossed. Contract your abs to curl your hips off the floor, reaching your legs up towards the ceiling, then lower your legs back down to their original position without letting your feet touch the floor. This ensures your abs are continually activated.

3. Janda sit-up

Lie on your back with your knees bent and hands placed behind your head. Then try 'digging' your heels into the floor, contracting your hamstrings, whilst performing an ordinary crunch.

4. The Jacknife

Place a mat on the floor, lie down on your back and extend your arms above your head. Simultaneously lift your arms and legs toward the ceiling, until your fingertips touch your toes, then return to your starting position.

5. The extended plank

Get into a press-up position, placing your hands around 10 inches in front of your shoulders, with the toes of your shoes placed against the floor. Hold this position with your back straight and try to continue to breathe as normal.

Bedtime: Drink 8oz of water before you go to bed

<u>Day 13 Paleo Challenge</u>

Wake up: Drink water right away. Recommended is 8oz.

Morning workout: Do 10 push-ups to get your blood flowing

Breakfast: 8oz of water and Egg Quiche

Ingredients:

12 eggs

Chopped vegetables

Chopped cooked meat

Splash of water (for fluffiness)

Salt & Pepper

You'll also need:

A pitcher

A non-stick muffin tin

Procedures:

1. Preheat oven to 350 degrees.

2. Chop a variety of vegetables such as spinach, broccoli, asparagus, roasted red peppers, mushrooms, sundried tomatoes, etc. Anything you have on hand will work.

3. If you choose to use meat, such as bacon, cook it first.

4. Break the eggs into a pitcher. Add a splash of water and season with salt and pepper. Mix well.

5. Pour a small amount of the egg mixture into the muffin tin (fill each about 1/3 full). Sprinkle the meat and vegetables of your choice into the tin and then cover with more egg mixture.

6. Cook for 15-20 minutes and then let them rest for 5 minutes before removing from the tin.

Drink 16oz of water by lunch time

Lunch: Roasted Beets

Servings: 4

Ingredients:

6 beets

1 tsp orange zest

2 tsp maple syrup

2 tbsp olive oil

½ cup balsamic vinegar

Sea salt and black pepper

Procedures:

1. Heat oven to 325 degrees
2. Slice beet into quarters and cut into thinner slices
3. Put beets on baking sheet, drizzle with olive oil and sprinkle with salt and pepper
4. Put in oven for 45 minutes
5. Put pan to high heat and put together vinegar and syrup
6. Remove from heat when mixture becomes a syrupy
7. Remove beets from oven and glaze syrup
8. Add the zest
9. Serve

Drink another 8oz of water after lunch.

Snack: Fruit Salad

Servings: 2

Ingredients:

1 apple, diced

1 orange, diced

½ cup pecans

½ cup walnuts

½ tsp cinnamon powder

Procedures:

1. Put fruits into bowl
2. Chop nuts into smaller pieces
3. Drizzle nuts in top of fruits
4. Sprinkle with cinnamon
5. Serve

Dinner: Paleo Teriyaki Salmon

Ingredients

Salmon:

4 fillets, about 6 ounces each - preferably wild-caught

Paleo Teriyaki Sauce:

1/2 cup coconut aminos

1/2 cup raw honey

1/4 cup juice from fresh oranges

2 tbs rice vinegar

1 tbs fresh grated ginger

1-2 garlic cloves, pressed or minced

1 tbs sesame oil

Pinch of red pepper flakes

Optional: Add 1 tsp arrowroot flour to make the sauce thicker

Directions

Teriyaki Sauce:

1. Combine all above teriyaki ingredients in a saucepan over medium heat

2. When mixture begins to boil, stir for another 2-3 minutes

3. Remove from heat and allow to cool

Salmon Prep:

1. Season with salt & pepper

2. Suggested: Use a portion of the teriyaki sauce to marinade fillets in refrigerator for one hour or more. Discard used marinade!

Grilling Method:

1. Place on medium high grill, skin side down

2. Grill for about 8-10 minutes, basting occasionally with fresh teriyaki sauce

3. Check often – grill just until sides are opaque and fish flakes easily with a fork.

Pan Sear/Baking Method:

1. Sear marinated fillets in hot skillet for just a few minutes until flesh is slightly charred

2. Place fillets in a baking dish, brush with teriyaki sauce, and bake at 350° F for about 10 minutes, or just until fish flakes easily

Garnish:

1. Sprinkle with sesame seeds or chopped green onions

Exercise of the day: Lateral Lunge Side Kick

Stand with feet together, arms at the sides and with 5-to 10-pound dumbbells in each hand. Step the right foot out to the side and bend the left knee at a 90-degree angle to come into a side lunge. Push into your left foot and come to standing with the knees slightly bent. Immediately kick the left foot strongly out to the side (make sure it stays flexed). Return to starting position.

Do 3 sets of 12-15 reps and repeat on the opposite side.

Bedtime: Drink 8oz of water before you go to bed

Day 14 Paleo Challenge

Last Day of the week! Push yourself harder today!

Wake up: Drink water right away. Recommended is 8oz.

Morning workout: Raise your calf with your feet turned out, feet straight and feet turned in. Do this 10 times each.

Breakfast: 8oz of water and Paleo Strawberry Crepes

Ingredients:

Crêpe Batter:

2 eggs whisked

1 cup of full-fat coconut milk (or you can use unsweetened almond milk)

1 tbs of olive oil

3/4 cup of tapioca flour

3 tbs of coconut flour

1/4 tsp sea salt

1 tsp pure vanilla

Crêpe Filling Ingredients:

2 lbs strawberries (or about 4 cups sliced) - divide in half

2 tbs lemon juice

3 tbs water

2 tbs raw honey

Procedures:

2. Cook the crêpes:

3. Follow the instructions for my Paleo Tortillas with the follow exceptions:

4. Don't forget to add the teaspoon of vanilla to the batter!

5. Lightly coat your skillet (or crêpe pan) with coconut oil over medium heat

6. When the pan is hot, ladle only 1/4 cup of crêpe batter into the center of the pan, then lift the skillet and tilt the pan with a circular motion to swirl the batter around the bottom to thin it out, then continue cooking the crêpe

7. Repeat the same process for each crêpe

Prepare the crêpe filling:

1. Clean, remove tops, and slice strawberries - you should have about 4 cups of sliced strawberries total

2. Place 2 cups of the sliced strawberries in a medium saucepan with lemon juice, water, and honey

3. Bring saucepan mixture to a boil, then reduce to medium heat for 20-30 minutes, stirring occasionally. When strawberries have cooked down into a sauce, remove from heat

4. While sauce is still warm, lightly stir in the remaining 2 cups of sliced strawberries and allow mixture to cool down a little

5. Fold and top the crêpes with about 1/4 cup each of the strawberry filling (as pictured) or place filling on a flat crêpe and roll up

6. Serve warm and enjoy!

Drink 16oz of water by lunch time

Lunch: Lettuce Combos

Servings: 2

Ingredients:

1 head lettuce

4 tbsp coconut aminos

2 tbsp ginger, grated

1 cup carrots cut into thin strips

8 oz. shitake mushrooms, sliced

1 cup bamboo shots, cut into thin strips

2 cloves garlic

1 tsp fish sauce

Sea salt and black pepper

Procedures:

1. Put skillet in medium heat and put oil
2. Put carrots, garlic, ginger, mushrooms and shoots in skillet and sauté for 2 minutes
3. Add fish sauce and cook for another 5 minutes
4. Remove from heat and set aside
5. Take one lettuce leaf and scoop in the veggie mixture into the lettuce. Wrap into a cone
6. Serve

Drink another 8oz of water after lunch.

Snack: Celery with 2 tablespoons of sunflower butter or baby carrots and few raisins.

Dinner: Slow-cooked Spicy Shredded Beef Tacos and 8oz of water

Ingredients:

Taco Ingredients:

2 lbs chuck roast

1/4 cup lime juice

3 tbs tomato paste

1/4 cup beef broth

1 medium onion, diced

1 serrano pepper, diced small

1 jalapeno pepper. diced small

3 garlic cloves, minced or pressed

1 tbs chili powder

1 tsp paprika

1/2 tsp cumin

1/2 tsp salt

1/2 tsp pepper

Procedures:

1. Season roast with salt and pepper and set aside

2. Mix dry spices together (chili powder, cumin, paprika) and rub over both sides of roast

3. Place roast in your slow cooker along with the garlic, onion and peppers

4. Combine remaining ingredients (tomato paste, beef stock, lime juice) and pour over beef

5. Cook on Low (8-10 hours) or High (4-6 hours) – meat should be tender and pull apart easily

6. Shred meat with a fork and return to slow cooker. Mix shredded meat with the juices remaining in the slow cooker

7. Make the paleo tortillas or use the shredded beef for a taco salad

8. Top as desired with the avocado cilantro lime sauce

Exercise of the day: 20 minute Killer Core Workout

As this is a longer workout, it is best that you follow the workout in the video below. Push yourself hard tonight as this is the last workout of the week! Drink plenty of water throughout the exercise.

Workout video → https://www.youtube.com/watch?v=KUjFh4J1dnc

Bedtime: Drink 8oz of water before you go to bed

Day 15 Paleo Challenge

Day 15 onwards is a repeated routine from week 1 and 2. You are free to follow or plan your own routines since you are now learning to live the Paleo life. You can do it!

Wake up: Drink water right away. Recommended is 8oz.

Morning workout: Raise your calf with your feet turned out, feet straight and feet turned in. Do this 10 times each.

Breakfast: Coco-Paleo Pancakes and 8oz of water

Yes, you can still have pancakes with the Paleo Diet by using coconut flour in your mixture.

Ingredients

3tbps. Coconut flour

¼ tsp. baking soda

3 medium-sized eggs

1 tbsp. coconut oil

3 tbsp. coconut milk

2 tbsp. apple sauce (unsweetened)

½ tsp. apple cider vinegar

Procedures:

4. In a bowl, mix the coconut flour and eggs until they are smooth. Add the applesauce, coconut oil, milk, baking soda, vinegar and a small amount of honey.

5. Heat a skillet over medium fire and drizzle hot coconut oil. When the pan is hot, add a small amount of the mixture. Cook the pancakes, until they turn golden brown.

6. Serve with blueberries or strawberries on top and drizzle with honey.

Drink 16oz of water before eating your lunch.

Lunch: Chicken and Avocado Salad Delight

Ingredients

2 boneless and skinless chicken breasts (cooked and cut into cubes)

1 large avocado (mashed)

2 tbsp. walnuts (chopped)

2 tbsp. fresh cilantro

1 freshly squeezed lime

Salt to taste

Procedures:

1. In a big bowl, combine the cubed chicken and mashed avocado.
2. Throw in the walnuts, finely chopped cilantro, lime juice, and add a pinch of salt to taste.
3. Combine ingredients thoroughly and serve.

Drink another 8oz of water after lunch.

Snack: Homemade Apple Chips

Get a quick sweet fix with these homemade apple chips.

Ingredients

2 pcs. Honeycrisp apple

1 tsp. cinnamon powder

1 tsp. raw honey

Procedures:

1. Preheat oven to 250°F.

2. Cut the apples in half and remove the seeds. Take a mandolin and slice the apples thinly.

3. Take a baking sheet and lay over with parchment paper.Take the apple slices and lay them separately. Sprinkle the cinnamon powder over the apple slices.

4. Place in the oven and cook or an hour. Flip the apples and cook for another 1 hour. Take out the oven and drizzle with honey.

5. Consume after cooling or store in an airtight container.

Dinner: Baked Salmon Dinner

This is a simple yet tasty baked salmon recipe.

Ingredients:

1 pc. Wild-caught salmon (32 oz.)

1 lemon (sliced thinly)

1 tbsp. capers

1 tbsp. thyme

Olive oil

Salt and pepper to taste

Procedures:

1. Pre-heat oven to 400°F

2. Prepare a baking sheet and top it with parchment paper. Place the salmon (skin side first) on the sheet and season with salt and pepper.

3. Top the salmon with capers, lemon and fresh thyme and bake in the oven for 25 minutes.

4. Best served, when hot.

Exercise of the day: The Pike

Lie face up with your legs straight, arms at your sides, palms facing down. Raise your legs and torso 45 degrees off the floor. (Your body should look like a "V".) Reach your hands alongside your legs as high as you can without rounding your back.

Start with one set of 8-12 rep. Once you can consistently get 15 reps, add another set.

Bedtime: Drink 16oz of water before you go to bed

Day 16 Paleo Challenge

Wake up: Drink water right away. Recommended is 8oz.

Morning workout: Do 10 push-ups to get your blood flowing

Breakfast: 8oz of water and Heavenly Ham n' Eggs

A simple two-ingredient recipe you'll want to eat, every morning!

Ingredients

4 slices of ham

2 eggs

(spices for flavor)

Procedures:

1. Preheat your oven to 400 °F

2. Prepare a muffin pan by greasing it with coconut oil.

3. Place two pieces of ham on top of each other in one muffin cup. Repeat with the next muffin cup.

4. Crack the egg on top of the ham

    a. *(Optional: add scallions, basil, etc. on your egg for more flavor)*

5. Bake for 15 minutes and serve.

Drink 16oz of water before eating your lunch.

Lunch: Veggie-bun Sandwich

Ingredients:

1 pc. red bell pepper

2 slices turkey ham

½ avocado (cut into strips)

1 pc. seaweed strips

Procedures:

1. Take the bell pepper and slice it in half and remove the seeds.

2. Take one piece of bell pepper and top it with the ham, seaweed, and avocado.

3. Top with the other half of the bell pepper and stick a toothpick in the center. Enjoy.

Drink another 8oz of water after lunch.

Snack: Celery with 2 tablespoons of sunflower butter or baby carrots and few raisins.

Dinner: Low-carb Paleo Patties and 8oz of water

Ingredients

16 oz. ground lean turkey

1 tsp. Paprika

½ tsp. coriander

1 tsp. powdered onion

a pinch of cayenne pepper

a pinch of salt

a pinch of ground pepper

2 pcs. green onions (chopped)

1 pc. tomato (sliced)

2 cups arugula

1 pc. avocado (sliced)

Procedures:

1. In a bowl, place the ground turkey and add the onion powder, salt, pepper, paprika, cayenne pepper, and green onions and combine everything.

2. Use your hands to form into burger patties.

3. Heat the grill and cook the burgers for 5 minutes, per side.

4. Place the cooked patties over the arugula, tomatoes, and avocado. Serve.

Exercise of the day: Tree-pose Yoga

This pose will have your abdominals working overtime to help you stay grounded on one leg.

Shift your weight onto your left leg. Draw your right knee into your chest, grab your ankle, and press the bottom of your right foot onto your left thigh. If you feel wobbly keep your hand on your ankle while it's pressed into your thigh. If you're finding your balance really easily, press your palms together in front of your chest. Brace your abdominals in tight to your spine, making sure you can still breathe easily. Find a focal point and focus your gaze while you hold the pose for 10 long, deep breaths. Repeat on the other leg.

Bedtime: Drink 8oz of water before you go to bed

Day 17 Paleo Challenge

Wake up: Drink water right away. Recommended is 8oz.

Morning workout: Raise your calf with your feet turned out, feet straight and feet turned in. Do this 10 times each.

Breakfast: Kale Breakfast Muffin and 8oz of water

Ingredients:

½ cup kale (finely chopped)

1/8 cup onion chives (finely chopped)

¼ cup almond milk

3 eggs

4 slices of smoked turkey

Pepper to taste

Procedures:

1. Preheat oven to 350 °F

2. In a mixing bowl, whisk together the eggs, kale, chives, almond milk and sprinkle with pepper to taste

3. Take a muffin pan and grease it with coconut oil. Fill the muffin cups with two slices of smoked turkey each and fill 2/3 of it with the kale mixture.

4. Bake for 30 minutes. Let it cool and serve.

Drink 16oz of water by lunch time.

Lunch: Cucumber Sandwich

Ingredients:

1 pc.cucumber

3 slices turkey breast slices (low sodium)

Dijon mustard

Garlic and herb spreadable

Procedures:

1. Take the cucumber and cut in half. Remove the seeds.
2. Spread the garlic and herb on cucumber.
3. Add lay the turkey slices on top and drizzle with Dijon mustard.
4. Sandwich with the other half of the cucumber.
5. Enjoy.

Drink another 8oz of water after lunch.

Snack: Berry-coconut Shake

Ingredients

8 pcs. frozen strawberries

1 cup coconut milk

1 tsp. honey

1 tsp. almond butter

2 pcs. fresh strawberries

Coconut shavings

Procedures:

1. Blend the strawberries, coconut milk, honey and almond butter.
2. Top with sliced fresh strawberries and coconut shavings.

Dinner: Slow-cooked Chicken Zing and 8oz of water

A zesty take on your favorite chicken!

Ingredients

48 oz. chicken legs (drumsticks)

1/3 cup fresh orange juice

2 tsp. orange zest

¼ cup raw honey

3 cloves garlic (minced)

1 tbsp. grated ginger

1 tbsp. coconut aminos

½ tbsp. balsamic vinegar

1 tsp. tomato paste

1 tbsp. sesame seeds

(optional) ½ tbsp. Sriracha sauce

green onions (chopped)

sesame seeds

Procedures:

1. Whisk all the ingredients in a bowl (except chicken).

2. Season the chicken with salt and pepper and place in a slow cooker and pour the sauce. Place in a slow cooker and cook over low heat for 4 hours.

3. Place the chicken on a plate and place the sauce in a small pan. Simmer the sauce for 15 minutes. Pour the sauce on the chicken and garnish with green onions and sesame seeds.

Exercise of the day: Side Plank

Lie on your left side with your elbow directly beneath your shoulder and legs stacked. Place your right hand on your left shoulder or on your right hip.

Brace your abs and lift your hips off the floor until you're balancing on your forearm and feet so that your body forms a diagonal line. Hold for 30 to 45 seconds. If you can't hold that long, stay up as long as you can and then repeat until you've held for 30 seconds total. Switch sides and repeat.

This abs exercise is more challenging than a traditional plank because you're supporting your entire body weight on two points of contact instead of four. As a result, you must work your core harder to stay stabilized.

Bedtime: Drink 8oz of water before you go to bed

Day 18 Paleo Challenge

Wake up: Drink water right away. Recommended is 8oz.

Morning workout: Do 10 push-ups to get your blood flowing

Breakfast: 8oz of water and Easy-o-whip Gluten-Free Banana Pancakes

Enjoy this delicious meal in just three easy steps!

Ingredients

¼ teaspoon baking powder

4 eggs

2 large bananas (chopped)

Procedures:

1. Place the ingredients in a bowl and mix with an immersion blender.

2. Heat a non-stick pan over medium-high heat.

3. Ladle the batter and place on the pan one at a time. Cook until the pancake bubbles, then flip and cook for another 30 seconds. Serve.

Drink 16oz of water before eating your lunch.

Lunch: Prosciutto Wrapped Chicken

A delicious and protein rich meal.

Ingredients:

3 pcs. chicken legs

1 tbsp. coconut oil

1 small shallot (chopped)

2 garlic cloves (minced)

2 cups spinach (frozen, roughly chopped)

1/3 cup olives (chopped)

3 slices prosciutto

1 tbsp. olive oil

salt and pepper to taste

Procedures:

1. Preheat oven to 325°F

2. Heat the pan over medium fire and drizzle with coconut oil.

3. Saute the garlic and shallots for 2 minutes.

4. Toss in the spinach and olives and cook for 5 minutes.

5. Remove from the heat and set in a bowl.

6. Top the mixture on the chicken thigh and wrap each leg with a slice of prosciutto.

7. Take a ceramic baking dish and drizzle with olive oil. Place the chicken on the dish and bake in he oven for an hour, or until the internal temperature reached 155°F.

Drink another 8oz of water after lunch.

Snack: Green Paleo Smoothie

This healthy and refreshing drink will not only quench your thirst but will also satisfy your cravings for sweets.

Ingredients

1 pc. mango (diced)

2 cups kale (stems removed)

½ lime (juiced)

1 pc. kiwi (diced)

1 cup coconut milk

water

Procedures:

1. Blend all the ingredients together, adding water to achieve your preferred consistency.

Dinner: Beef Skewers and 8oz of water

Start the grill and cook these beef kebabs for dinner!

Ingredients:

32 oz. sirloin beef (cut into 2" cubes)

1 pc. zucchini (cut into 1" cubes)

1 onion (cut into 1" squares)

1 red or green bell pepper (cut into 1" squares)

Marinade

5 garlic cloves

1 small onion (chopped)

¼ cup squeezed orange juice

1 tsp. orange zest

1 tbsp. rosemary (chopped)

¼ cup olive oil

2 tbsp. organic tomato paste

sea salt and pepper to taste

Procedures:

2. Combine all the marinade recipes in a food processor until you reach a smooth paste. Set aside ¼ cup of the marinade for the veggies.

3. In a bowl, place beef and pour over the marinade. Toss the beef to make sure that it is well-coated with the marinade. Refrigerate it overnight.

4. When you're ready to cook, remove the beef in the fridge 30 minutes before grilling, to allow it to thaw.

5. Take the ¼ cup marinade and toss it with the vegetables in a bowl.

6. Thread the beef cubes and vegetables alternately using bamboo or metal skewers.

7. Bring the grill over medium heat and cook the kebabs, turning each side after four minutes. The whole kebab will cook in about 12 minutes or until it is well-cooked.

Exercise of the day: Walkout from Pushup Position

Start in a pushup position with your hands two inches wider than your shoulders.

Walk hands out as far as possible, then walk back. Do 10-12 reps.

Bedtime: Drink 8oz of water before you go to bed

Day 19 Paleo Challenge

Wake up: Drink water right away. Recommended is 8oz.

Morning workout: Raise your calf with your feet turned out, feet straight and feet turned in. Do this 10 times each.

Breakfast: 8oz of water and Paleo-friendly Banana Loaf

Who says you can't eat bread when you go Paleo? Try this Paleo-friendly recipe for a breakfast loaf!

Ingredients:

4 large bananas (mashed)

4 tbsp. Coconut oil (or grass-fed butter)

4 eggs

½ cup almond flour (you can also use coconut flour as a substitute)

1 tsp. baking soda

1 tsp. gluten-free baking powder

1 tsp. cinnamon powder

½ cup almond butter

1 tsp. vanilla extract

a pinch of sea salt

Procedures:

1. Preheat oven to 350°F

2. In a bowl, mix the bananas, eggs, and coconut oil and blend well using a hand mixer.

3. Once all the ingredients are well-blended, add the almond flour, cinnamon, baking powder, baking soda, vanilla and sea salt. Mix well.

4. Grease a loaf pan and pour the batter. Cook in the oven for an hour, until its color, turns golden brown.

5. Flip the cooked loaf on a cooling rack. Slice and serve.

Drink 16oz of water before eating your lunch.

Lunch: Perfect Paleo Meatloaf

This is a perfect Paleo-friendly meatloaf you can cook, especially on Sunday dinners.

Ingredients

32 oz. lean, organic pork (ground)

10 oz. thawed frozen spinach (squeeze excess water)

1 onion (diced)

6 oz. mushrooms (diced)

2 pcs. carrots (diced)

4 eggs (beaten)

2 tsp. olive oil

2 tsp. sea salt

2 tsp. freshly ground pepper

2 tsp. onion powder

1 tsp. thyme

1 tsp. garlic powder

1/3 cup coconut flour

¼ tsp. grated nutmeg

Procedures:

1. Preheat oven at 375°F

2. Place a pan on medium fire and drizzle with olive oil. Saute the onions and mushrooms, until the onions are caramelized. Remove from the heat and let it cool.

3. In a large bowl, combine the meat, chopped spinach, cooked onions and mushrooms, eggs, spices and coconut flour. Mix well with your hands, making sure to break up the meat.

4. Grease a loaf pan and fill with the meat mixture.

5. Cook in the oven for about 25 minutes, or until the internal temperature reaches 160°F.

6. After cooking, remove from the oven and let it cool before serving.

Drink another 8oz of water after lunch.

Snack: Homemade Apple Chips (repeat day one snack)

Get a quick sweet fix with these homemade apple chips.

Ingredients:

2 pcs. Honeycrisp apple

1 tsp. cinnamon powder

1 tsp. raw honey

Procedures:

1. Preheat oven to 250°F.

2. Cut the apples in half and remove the seeds. Take a mandolin and slice the apples thinly.

3. Take a baking sheet and lay over with parchment paper.Take the apple slices and lay them separately. Sprinkle the cinnamon powder over the apple slices.

4. Place in the oven and cook or an hour. Flip the apples and cook for another 1 hour. Take out the oven and drizzle with honey.

Consume after cooling or store in an airtight container.

Dinner: Grilled Pork Chops with Pear Relish and 8oz of water

This meaty, fruity combo is a recipe you'll enjoy eating!

Ingredients:

2 pcs. pork chops

¼ cup mustard

1 cup pear (pitted and diced)

1 small shallot (diced)

1/8 cup fresh basil (finely chopped)

1 ½ tbsp. apple cider vinegar

1/8 cup olive oil

Procedures:

1. Marinate pork chops in a salt and pepper rub for 30 mins.

2. In a mixing bowl, combine the mustard, pear, diced shallot, basil, vinegar, olive oil and set aside.

3. When marinated, place the chops on a preheated grill and cook for six minutes each side.

4. Serve pork chops with peach relish on top.

Exercise of the day: The Pike

Lie face up with your legs straight, arms at your sides, palms facing down. Raise your legs and torso 45 degrees off the floor. (Your body should look like a "V".) Reach your hands alongside your legs as high as you can without rounding your back.

Start with one set of 8-12 rep. Once you can consistently get 15 reps, add another set.

Bedtime: Drink 8oz of water before you go to bed

Day 20 Paleo Challenge

Wake up: Drink water right away. Recommended is 8oz.

Morning workout: Do 10 push-ups to get your blood flowing

Breakfast: 8oz of water and Homemade Corned Beef

Have corned beef and radishes (instead of potatoes) with this recipe!

Ingredients:

2 cups corned beef (cooked and chopped)

3 cups radishes (cut into quarters)

1 small onion (chopped)

2 garlic cloves (minced)

½ cup beef broth

salt and pepper to taste

Procedures:

1. Heat a pan over medium-high heat and drizzle with oil.

2. Saute the onions for 4 minutes and then add radishes. Cook for another 5 minutes.

3. Add the garlic and sauté for another minute.

4. Pour in the broth and then cover loosely. Let it simmer for five minutes or until the radishes are tender.

5. Add the corned beef and stir well.

6. Season with a dash of salt and pepper.

Drink 16oz of water by lunch time.

Lunch: Chicken Salad

Servings: 2

Ingredients:

2 chicken breasts, skinned and deboned

1 avocado

2 tbsp cilantro

2 tbsp avocado

3 tbsp lime juice

1 tbsp coconut oil

sea salt

Procedures:

1. Heat pan to high and put oil, cook chicken. When cooked, cut chicken into small cubes
2. Place chicken in salad bowl and add rest of the ingredients
3. Add salt to taste
4. Serve

Drink another 8oz of water after lunch.

Snack: Apple with sunflower butter

Dinner: Seared Steak and 8oz of water

Servings: 2

Ingredients:

2 rib eye steaks

1 tbsp of rosemary

1 tbsp butter

1/4 tsp garlic powder

1/4 tsp onion powder

1/4 tsp paprika

1 tbsp coconut oil

5 cloves garlic

sea salt and black pepper

Procedures:

1. Create the steak rub by combining the garlic, onion and paprika powder with salt. Set aside when combined.
2. Heat pan on high for 2 minutes
3. Rub the oil into the steaks
4. Take steak rub and sprinkle on the steak
5. Put steak on pan and cook for 3 minutes on each side
6. Remove steak and put on plate
7. Lower the heat of pan and put rosemary, garlic and butter
8. Cook for 2 minutes, stir occasionally
9. Drip the butter mixture on the steaks
10. Serve

Exercise of the day: Warrior III

This yoga move can tone your legs, and core too.

Stand with the feet together, and lift up the left leg with a pointed toe, putting your body weight onto the standing, right leg. Continue to lift your leg and drop the head and torso so they form a straight horizontal line from head to toe with the arms at your sides. Engage your core and make sure the left thigh, hip, and toes are aligned. Remain facing down and keep your back as straight as possible. Ensure your right knee doesn't lock and center the weight on the middle of the foot. Hold for 5 breaths and then slowly return to standing.

Switch legs and repeat.

Bedtime: Drink 8oz of water before you go to bed

Day 21 Paleo Challenge

Wake up: Drink water right away. Recommended is 8oz.

Morning workout: Raise your calf with your feet turned out, feet straight and feet turned in. Do this 10 times each.

Breakfast: 8oz of water and Banana-berry Toast

Have this sweet and filling breakfast to jumpstart your day!

Ingredients:

1 loaf Paleo banana bread (refer to recipe 5)

1 cup blueberries (frozen)

1 cup coconut milk

5 eggs

¼ cup raw honey

1 tsp. vanilla extract

1 tsp. ground cinnamon

Procedures:

1. Preheat oven at 350°F
2. Cut the loaf into cubes and place in a baking dish (8x8") with the blueberries
3. In a mixing bowl, blend the coconut milk, honey, cinnamon, vanilla, and eggs.
4. Pour the mixture over the bread and berries and bake for 45 minutes.
5. When cooked, remove from the oven and allow to cool for 15 minutes. Serve.

Drink 16oz of water by lunch time

Lunch: Salmon Glaze

Servings: 2

Ingredients:

12 oz. salmon fillets

2 tbsp honey

1 tbsp coconut oil

2 tbsp coconut aminos

1 tbsp apple cider vinegar

1 tbsp grated ginger

1 tsp sesame seeds

1/2 tsp lime juice

1 tbsp chopped cilantro

Procedures:

1. Heat oven to 400 degrees
2. In a bowl, combine aminos, vinegar, honey and lime juice. Set aside.
3. Heat pan to high and put coconut oil
4. Sear salmon with the skin side of the fillet up until brown
5. When brown, flip salmon and drizzle honey glaze
6. Bake for 5 minutes
7. Remove and drizzle again with honey
8. Add garnishes, cilantro and seeds
9. Serve

Drink another 8oz of water after lunch.

Snack: Energy Bars

Servings: 5 bars

Ingredients:

•1 medium, banana (very ripe works best)

- 1/4 cup nuts (I used salted cashews)

- 1/3 cup dried fruit (I used cherries)

- 1/4 cup seeds (I used sunflower seeds, or sub for more nuts)

- 1/4 cup vanilla protein powder (try with another flavor and let me know how it is)

- 2 tbsp arrowroot starch (or other starch)

- 1/2 cup almond flour (thought I should add parenthesis here too)

Procedures:

1. In a bowl, mash the banana well with a fork or other handy utensil. It doesn't have to be perfect.

2. Add almond flour and arrowroot starch and mix well.

3. Add in your mix-ins and stir well.

4. Grease a small pan (I used a meatloaf pan and it was perfect) with your favorite oil and pour mixture in, pressing down where needed to evenly distribute throughout.

5. Bake on around 275 for 30-40 minutes, or until the edges start to brown.

6. Take out the loaf, and cut into cute bars or squares.

7. Power up as needed! And store in the fridge after a day.

Dinner: Thai Chicken and 8oz of water

Servings: 4

Ingredients:

1 lb. chicken breasts deboned and skinned

12 lettuce leaves

3 onions, sliced

1 carrot, shredded

1 broccoli, cut into florets

¼ cup cilantro

2 tbsp coconut aminos

2 tbsp lime juice

Water

Procedures:

1. Cook chicken and cut into small cubes
2. Take lettuce and spread on flat surface
3. Add chicken, carrots, cilantro and onions
4. Drizzle with aminos and lime juice
5. Serve

Exercise of the day: 20 minutes Killer Core Workout

As this is a longer workout, it is recommended that you follow the workout in the video below. Push yourself hard tonight as this is the last workout of the week! Drink plenty of water throughout the exercise.

Workout video → https://www.youtube.com/watch?v=KUjFh4J1dnc

Bedtime: Drink 8oz of water before you go to bed

Day 22 Paleo Challenge

Wake up: Drink water right away. Recommended is 8oz.

Morning workout: Do 10 push-ups to get your blood flowing

Breakfast: 8oz of water and Egg Muffin

Servings: 2

Ingredients:

1 cup lean meat, cooked and shredded

9 eggs

1 tsp paprika

3 tbsp coconut milk

1/2 cup tomatoes

1 onion, minced

1 tbsp coconut oil

sea salt and black pepper

Procedures:

1. Heat oven to 350 degrees
2. Heat pan on medium and put oil
3. Sauté onions for 5 minutes
4. Turn off heat and add meat. Set aside
5. Use a bowl and put together milk, eggs, salt, and pepper. Set aside
6. Put liners in muffin tin and add egg mixture
7. Add pinch paprika on top of each muffin
8. Place in oven and cook for 30 minutes
9. Serve

Drink 16oz of water by lunch time.

Lunch: Beef & Noodles

Servings: 3

Ingredients:

1/4 lb. flank steak cubed

1/2 pack squash noodles

1 egg scrambled and sliced into thin pieces

1/2 tbsp coconut oil

2 tbsp coconut aminos

1/4 cup bone broth

1 cup spinach

1/2 cup carrots, shredded

1/4 onion, sliced

2 cloves garlic, minced

1 stalk of green onion

1/2 tbsp sesame oil

1/2 tbsp sesame seeds

1/2 tsp fish sauce

1/2 pack mushrooms

Procedures:

1. Submerge spinach in boiling water and drain as soon as possible, completely dry by patting with paper towel. Mix sesame oil. Set aside and let cool.
2. Sauté garlic and onion in coconut oil add steak and cook until brown
3. Put in aminos, broth, carrots, mushrooms, eggs and fish sauce
4. Allow broth to simmer
5. Add noodles and stir occasionally
6. Cover and allow noodles to absorb the broth
7. Remove from heat and add the onions, spinach, and seeds
8. Serve

Drink another 8oz of water after lunch.

Snack: Celery with 2 tablespoons of sunflower butter or baby carrots and few raisins.

Dinner: Mackerel with Cabbage and 8oz of water

Servings: 5

Ingredients:

4 mackerel fillets

1 egg

3 tbsp olive oil

1/2 cup almond flour

1/4 tsp mustard powder

sea salt and black pepper

1 head cabbage

6 cloves garlic

2 cups broccoli florets

1 cup chicken broth

1 tbsp coconut oil

Procedures:

For the fish:

1. Heat oven to 350 degrees
2. Whisk egg and set aside
3. Use a plate and put together flour, mustard, salt, and pepper
4. Dip mackerel in egg and then in flour mixture
5. Heat skillet to medium, put oil and fry for 2 minutes
6. Place in oven for 10 minutes

For the cabbage:

1. Heat skillet to medium and put oil
2. Sauté garlic until fragrant and add cabbage, stir again
3. Add florets and cook for 1 minute
4. Pour broth and bring to a simmer
5. Take out fish from oven and put in plate
6. Put cabbage in small bowl and serve as a side

Exercise of the day: The Pike

Lie face up with your legs straight, arms at your sides, palms facing down. Raise your legs and torso 45 degrees off the floor. (Your body should look like a "V".) Reach your hands alongside your legs as high as you can without rounding your back.

Start with one set of 8-12 rep. Once you can consistently get 15 reps, add another set.

Bedtime: Drink 8oz of water before you go to bed

Day 23 Paleo Challenge

Wake up: Drink water right away. Recommended is 8oz.

Morning workout: Raise your calf with your feet turned out, feet straight and feet turned in. Do this 10 times each.

Breakfast: 8oz of water and Paleo Breakfast

Servings: 6

Ingredients:

3/4 lb. steak, slice into small pieces

4 eggs

2 sweet potatoes, chop into cubes

1 red bell pepper, chopped

1 green bell pepper, chopped

1 tomato, diced

2 tbsp. coconut oil

sea salt and black pepper to taste

Procedures:

1. Pre-heat oven to 350 degrees
2. Put oil in skillet and set to high
3. Place steak, cook until brown and then set aside
4. Sauté peppers and onions for 5 minutes
5. Add potatoes and cook for 10 minutes
6. Add steak and combine ingredients together
7. Use a spoon and dig small scoops in the potato mixture
8. Crack the eggs into the scoops
9. Put tomatoes on top of the eggs
10. Add salt and pepper to taste
11. Bake for 10 minutes

Drink 16oz of water by lunch time.

Lunch: Spaghetti & Sausage

Servings: 4

Ingredients:

4 Italian sausages

1 squash

8 oz. tomato sauce, organic

2 tbsp olive oil

2 tsp oregano

2 tsp basil

2 tsp thyme

6 clove garlic

Procedures:

1. Put oil, herbs, garlic and sauce on slow cooker and set to high
2. Halve the squash and remove the seeds
3. Add squash on stove and put on slow cooker
4. Cut sausages into small pieces and add to cooker. Leave for 3 hours
5. Take squash from stove and scrape flesh using fork; this creates the pasta
6. Put pasta on plate and top with the sauce
7. Serve

Drink another 8oz of water after lunch.

Snack: Berry-coconut Shake

Ingredients:

8 pcs. frozen strawberries

1 cup coconut milk

1 tsp. honey

1 tsp. almond butter

2 pcs. fresh strawberries

Coconut shavings

Procedures:

1. Blend the strawberries, coconut milk, honey and almond butter.

2. Top with sliced fresh strawberries and coconut shavings.

Dinner: Snapper

Servings: 4

Ingredients:

1 lb. red snapper fillet

1 bell pepper, chopped

¼ cup cilantro

1 onion, cut into thin slices

1 tomato, chopped

1 tbsp lemon juice

1 tbsp lime juice

1 tsp chili powder

Black pepper

Procedures:

1. Heat oven to 350 degrees

2. Put fish on baking dish
3. Drizzle lime and lemon juice and sprinkle chili powder
4. Leave for 10 minutes, turn every few minutes
5. Chop onions, peppers and tomato and sprinkle on top of fish
6. Cover and put in oven for 30 minutes
7. Allow 5 minutes outside the oven
8. Garnish with cilantro
9. Serve

Exercise of the day: Single Leg Lift and Row

This move works more than just the legs; it targets the back, arms, and core in addition to the butt and hamstrings.

Begin standing with your left foot in front of the right foot. Hold a 5- to 8-pound dumbbell in the right hand and keep both arms at your sides. Leaning forward, raise the right foot off the ground and bring it straight up to hip level. At the same time, bring the weight toward the ground and then raise it up to hip-level.

Do 12-15 reps on the right side before switching arms and legs to repeat on the left side.

Bedtime: Drink 8oz of water before you go to bed

Day 24 Paleo Challenge

Wake up: Drink water right away. Recommended is 8oz.

Morning workout: Do 10 push-ups to get your blood flowing

Breakfast: 8oz of water and Old Fashioned Pancakes

Servings: 2

Ingredients:

3 eggs

4 bananas

1/4 cup almond butter

1 tbsp coconut oil

Procedures:

1. Put banana and eggs in a bowl and mash together until smooth
2. Add butter, mix again until creamy
3. Put pan on heat and heat oil
4. Pour batter and cook until golden brown

Drink 16oz of water by lunch time.

Lunch: Turkey Sandwich

Servings: 2

Ingredients:

6 slices of turkey breast, cooked

1 cucumber

1 tbsp Dijon mustard

1 tsp garlic powder

1 tsp red pepper flakes

2 tbsp low-fat mayonnaise

Procedures:

1. Remove cucumber seeds and cut into small pieces and set aside
2. Make the spread by putting together garlic powder, pepper flakes and mayonnaise. Spread on the cucumber slices.
3. Put turkey slices and spread mustard on top
4. Serve

Drink another 8oz of water after lunch.

Snack: Green Paleo Smoothie

This healthy and refreshing drink will not only quench your thirst but will also satisfy your cravings for sweets.

Ingredients:

1 pc. mango (diced)

2 cups kale (stems removed)

½ lime (juiced)

1 pc. kiwi (diced)

1 cup coconut milk

water

Procedures:

1. Blend all the ingredients together, adding water to achieve your preferred consistency.

Dinner: Shrimp & Cauliflower

Servings: 2

Ingredients:

1/2 lb shrimp, remove vein and shell

1 head cauliflower

1/2 cup peas

1/2 cup carrots, chopped into thin slices

1 yellow squash, chopped

1 bell pepper, chopped

1/4 tsp red pepper flakes

1 tbsp minced ginger

1 tsp coconut oil

sea salt and black pepper

Procedures:

2. Grate cauliflower into a rice-like consistency
3. Put skillet on medium heat, put oil. Sauté onion and garlic
4. Add cauliflower, salt and pepper. Cook for 5 minutes and set aside
5. Put oil and add pepper flakes, garlic and ginger and cook for 2 minutes
6. Add carrots, bell pepper, peas and squash and fry until bright in color and set aside
7. Put oil and add shrimp and ginger, fry until shrimp is pink
8. Add vegetables for 2 minutes
9. Add cauliflower rice and stir for 2 minutes
10. Serve

Exercise of the day: 10 minutes routine (repeat 3 times)

1. The long-arm crunch 12 reps
2. Reverse crunch 12 reps
3. Janda sit-up 12 reps
4. The Jackknife 12 reps

5. Extended Plank 45 seconds

1. The long-arm crunch

Do a traditional crunch by lying on your back with your arms straightened and your knees bent. Keep your arms straight above your head and make sure that the movement is controlled and at a moderate pace.

2. The reverse crunch

Lie on your back and place your hands behind your head, then bring your knees in towards your chest until they're bent to 90 degrees, with feet together or crossed. Contract your abs to curl your hips off the floor, reaching your legs up towards the ceiling, then lower your legs back down to their original position without letting your feet touch the floor. This ensures your abs are continually activated.

3. Janda sit-up

Lie on your back with your knees bent and hands placed behind your head. Then try 'digging' your heels into the floor, contracting your hamstrings, while performing an ordinary crunch.

4. The Jackknife

Place a mat on the floor, lie down on your back and extend your arms above your head. Simultaneously lift your arms and legs toward the ceiling, until your fingertips touch your toes, then return to your starting position.

5. The extended plank

Get into a press-up position, placing your hands around 10 inches in front of your shoulders, with the toes of your shoes placed against the floor. Hold this position with your back straight and try to continue to breathe as normal.

Bedtime: Drink 8oz of water before you go to bed

Day 25 Paleo Challenge

Wake up: Drink water right away. Recommended is 8oz.

Morning workout: Do 10 push-ups to get your blood flowing

Breakfast: 8oz of water and Egg Breakfast

Servings: 2

Ingredients:

2 eggs

1 tbsp coconut oil

1 cup spinach, chopped

1 cup broccoli flowers, cooked

1/2 avocado, cut into small chunks

1 /2 cup tomatoes cut into small sizes

sea salt and black pepper

Procedures:

1. Heat pan on low and put coconut oil
2. Cook sunny side eggs
3. Put vegetable ingredients, except avocado, on bowl and toss
4. Put eggs on top of vegetables
5. Add salt and pepper to taste
6. Top with avocado
7. Serve

Drink 16oz of water by lunch time.

Lunch: Spinach and Pancetta Frittatas

Servings: 4 - 6

Ingredients:

6 eggs

1/3 cup coconut milk

3 oz diced pancetta

1/2 cup diced onion

2 cups shredded raw sweet potato

2 cups fresh spinach leaves

salt, pepper, any other favorite seasonings

Procedures:

1. In a mixing bowl, whisk the eggs
2. Add the coconut milk, salt, pepper, any other herbs or seasoning you like. Stir and set aside.
3. Preheat oven to 350° F
4. Brown the pancetta over medium heat on an oven-proof frying pan. When browned, remove pancetta but leave the fat in frying pan
5. Add the onions and shredded sweet potatoes – cook in the pancetta fat for about 3 minutes
6. Add spinach to frying pan and cook until leaves start to wilt
7. Now take your bowl of whisked eggs and pour over the potatoes, onions and spinach in the frying pan
8. Allow to cook for about 2 minutes, then sprinkle the pancetta on top
9. Transfer the pan to the preheated 350° F oven and bake for 20-25 minutes until cooked through
10. Remove from oven and allow it to rest for a minute or two
11. Slice and serve!

Note: You may use fried and chopped bacon strips if pancetta is unavailable

Drink another 8oz of water after lunch.

Snack: Apple with sunflower butter

Dinner: Fish Sticks and 8oz of water

Servings: 12 sticks

Ingredients:

1/2 lb cream dory fillets

2 eggs

1 tbsp coconut oil

2 cups almond flour

sea salt and black pepper

Procedures:

1. Put eggs in bowl and whisk
2. Use bowl and put together flour, salt and pepper
3. Heat skillet to medium and put in oil
4. Cut fillets into thin strips, dip in egg mixture and then in flour
5. Fry for 2 minutes
6. Remove fish sticks and put in paper towel
7. Serve

Exercise of the day: Rock 'n Roll Lotus

Sit with your legs crossed at the ankles. Hold onto the outside of each ankle with your opposite hand, and lift your legs off the floor, balancing on your sitting bones. Pull your abs into your spine and take a deep breath in. As you exhale, begin to round onto your back. Continue rolling until your shoulder blades touch the floor, lifting your hips, still holding onto your ankles. Keeping your abs in tight, rock back up to sitting, finding your balance again on your sitting bones. That's one rep. Repeat 10 times.

Imagine you are using your abs as brakes to help you stop at the top and bottom of the rocking motion.

Bedtime: Drink 8oz of water before you go to bed

Day 26 Paleo Challenge

Wake up: Drink water right away. Recommended is 8oz.

Morning workout: Raise your calf with your feet turned out, feet straight and feet turned in. Do this 10 times each.

Breakfast: 8oz of water and Paleo Blueberry Muffin

Ingredients:

2 1/2 cups almond meal (almond flour)

3 large eggs, fresh

1/2 cups Cooper's pure raw honey

1/2 tsp baking powder

1/2 tsp salt

1 tbsp vanilla extract

1 cup blueberries, fresh

Procedures:

1. Preheat oven to 300°.
2. Line a 6 cup muffin pan with muffin liners.
3. In a large bowl, mix all ingredients together, except blueberries, until full combined. Gently fold in blueberries.
4. Fill each liner 3/4 full with batter.
5. Bake for 30-40 minutes. (Top should be spongy, but firm when pressed.)
6. Cool for 5 minutes and remove from muffin pan.

Drink 16oz of water by lunch time.

Lunch: Vegan Salad

Servings: 2

Ingredients:

2 cups mushrooms

2 cups cucumber, sliced

2 cups spinach, chopped

2 cups lettuce, torn

1/4 cup carrot, sliced

1/4 cup cucumber, sliced

1/4 cup onion, sliced

1 tbsp coconut oil

1 tbsp olive oil

Procedures:

1. Put skillet on high heat and put coconut oil
2. Sauté onion, garlic, mushrooms and spinach for 5 minute and set aside
3. Toss remaining ingredients, except olive oil, in bowl
4. Take the tossed ingredients and sautéed vegetables and put together
5. Drizzle with olive oil
6. Serve

Drink another 8oz of water after lunch.

Snack: Celery with 2 tablespoons of sunflower butter or baby carrots and few raisins.

Dinner: Chicken Pesto

Servings: 2

Ingredients:

2 chicken breasts

1/2 cup basil leaves

1/3 cup walnuts, chopped

2 cloves garlic

1 tsp rosemary leaves, dried

2 tbsp EVOO

sea salt and black pepper

Procedures:

1. Heat oven to 375 degrees
2. Put basil, garlic, walnuts and oil in a food process, blend until pasty texture
3. Create a flap on the chicken breast and use heavy object to flatten the breast
4. Stuff pesto paste in breast, reseals with the flap
5. Put salt and pepper to taste and bake for 30 minutes
6. Serve

Exercise of the day: 10 minutes routine (repeat 3 times)

1. The long-arm crunch 12 reps
2. Reverse crunch 12 reps
3. Janda sit-up 12 reps
4. The Jackknife 12 reps
5. Extended Plank 45 seconds

1. The long-arm crunch

Lie on your back with your knees bent and your arms straightened behind you. Then, keeping your arms straight above your head, perform a traditional crunch. The movement should be slow and controlled.

2. The reverse crunch

Lie on your back and place your hands behind your head, then bring your knees in towards your chest until they're bent to 90 degrees, with feet together or crossed.

Contract your abs to curl your hips off the floor, reaching your legs up towards the ceiling, then lower your legs back down to their original position without letting your feet touch the floor. This ensures your abs are continually activated.

3. Janda sit-up

Lie on your back with your knees bent and hands placed behind your head. Then try 'digging' your heels into the floor, contracting your hamstrings, while performing an ordinary crunch.

4. The Jackknife

Place a mat on the floor, lie down on your back and extend your arms above your head. Simultaneously lift your arms and legs toward the ceiling, until your fingertips touch your toes, then return to your starting position.

5. The extended plank

Get into a press-up position, placing your hands around 10 inches in front of your shoulders, with the toes of your shoes placed against the floor. Hold this position with your back straight and try to continue to breathe as normal.

Bedtime: Drink 8oz of water before you go to bed

Day 27 Paleo Challenge

Wake up: Drink water right away. Recommended is 8oz.

Morning workout: Do 10 push-ups to get your blood flowing

Breakfast: 8oz of water and Egg Quiche

Ingredients:

12 eggs

Chopped vegetables

Chopped cooked meat

Splash of water (for fluffiness)

Salt & Pepper

You'll also need:

A pitcher

A non-stick muffin tin

Procedures:

1. Preheat oven to 350 degrees.

2. Chop a variety of vegetables such as spinach, broccoli, asparagus, roasted red peppers, mushrooms, sundried tomatoes, etc. Anything you have on hand will work.

3. If you choose to use meat, such as bacon, cook it first.

4. Break the eggs into a pitcher. Add a splash of water and season with salt and pepper.

5. Mix well.

6. Pour a small amount of the egg mixture into the muffin tin (fill each about 1/3 full). Sprinkle the meat and vegetables of your choice into the tin and then cover with more egg mixture.

7. Cook for 15-20 minutes and then let them rest for 5 minutes before removing from the tin.

Drink 16oz of water by lunch time

Lunch: Roasted Beets

Servings: 4

Ingredients:

6 beets

1 tsp orange zest

2 tsp maple syrup

2 tbsp olive oil

½ cup balsamic vinegar

Sea salt and black pepper

Procedures:
1. Heat oven to 325 degrees
2. Slice beet into quarters and cut into thinner slices
3. Put beets on baking sheet, drizzle with olive oil and sprinkle with salt and pepper
4. Put in oven for 45 minutes
5. Put pan to high heat and put together vinegar and syrup
6. Remove from heat when mixture becomes a syrupy
7. Remove beets from oven and glaze syrup
8. Add the zest
9. Serve

Drink another 8oz of water after lunch.

Snack: Fruit Salad

Servings: 2

Ingredients:

1 apple, diced

1 orange, diced

½ cup pecans

½ cup walnuts

½ tsp cinnamon powder

Procedures:

1. Put fruits into bowl
2. Chop nuts into smaller pieces
3. Drizzle nuts on top of fruits
4. Sprinkle with cinnamon
5. Serve

Dinner: Paleo Teriyaki Salmon

Ingredients

Salmon:

4 fillets, about 6 ounces each - preferably wild-caught

Paleo Teriyaki Sauce:

1/2 cup coconut aminos

1/2 cup raw honey

1/4 cup juice from fresh oranges

2 tbs rice vinegar

1 tbs grated fresh ginger

1-2 garlic cloves, pressed or minced

1 tbs sesame oil

Pinch of red pepper flakes

Optional: Add 1 tsp arrowroot flour to make the sauce thicker

Procedures:

Teriyaki Sauce:

1. Combine all above teriyaki ingredients in a saucepan over medium heat

2. When mixture begins to boil, stir for another 2-3 minutes

3. Remove from heat and allow to cool

Salmon Prep:

Season with salt & pepper

Suggested: Use a portion of the teriyaki sauce to marinade fillets in the refrigerator for one hour or more. Discard used marinade!

Grilling Method:

1. Place on medium high grill, skin side down

2. Grill for about 8-10 minutes, occasionally basting with fresh teriyaki sauce

3. Check often – grill just until sides are opaque and fish flakes easily with a fork.

Pan Sear/Baking Method:

1. Sear marinated fillets in hot skillet for just a few minutes until flesh is slightly charred

2. Place fillets in a baking dish, brush with teriyaki sauce, and bake at 350° F for about 10 minutes, or just until fish flakes easily

Garnish:

Sprinkle with sesame seeds or chopped green onions

Exercise of the day: Lateral Lunge Side Kick

Stand with feet together, arms at the sides and with 5-to 10-pound dumbbells in each hand. Step the right foot out to the side and bend the left knee at a 90-degree angle to come into a side lunge. Push into your left foot and come to standing with the knees slightly bent. Immediately kick the left foot strongly out to the side (make sure it stays flexed). Return to starting position.

Do 3 sets of 12-15 reps and repeat on the opposite side.

Bedtime: Drink 8oz of water before you go to bed

Day 28 Paleo Challenge

Last Day of the week! Push yourself harder today!

Wake up: Drink water right away. Recommended is 8oz.

Morning workout: Raise your calf with your feet turned out, feet straight and feet turned in. Do this 10 times each.

Breakfast: 8oz of water and Paleo Strawberry Crepes

Ingredients:

Crêpe Batter:

2 eggs whisked

1 cup of full-fat coconut milk (or you can use unsweetened almond milk)

1 tbs of olive oil

3/4 cup of tapioca flour

3 tbs of coconut flour

1/4 tsp sea salt

1 tsp pure vanilla

Crêpe Filling Ingredients:

2 lbs strawberries (or about 4 cups sliced) - divide in half

2 tbs lemon juice

3 tbs water

2 tbs raw honey

Procedures:

1. Cook the crêpes:

2. Follow the instructions for my Paleo Tortillas with the follow exceptions:

3. Don't forget to add the teaspoon of vanilla to the batter!

4. Lightly coat your skillet (or crêpe pan) with coconut oil over medium heat

5. When the pan is hot, ladle only 1/4 cup of crêpe batter into the center of the pan, then lift the skillet and tilt the pan with a circular motion to swirl the batter around the bottom to thin it out, then continue cooking the crêpe

6. Repeat the same process for each crêpe

Prepare the crêpe filling:

1. Clean, remove tops, and slice strawberries - you should have about 4 cups of sliced strawberries total

2. Place 2 cups of the sliced strawberries in a medium saucepan with lemon juice, water, and honey

3. Bring saucepan mixture to a boil, then reduce to medium heat for 20-30 minutes, stirring occasionally. When strawberries have cooked down into a sauce, remove from heat

4. While sauce is still warm, lightly stir in the remaining 2 cups of sliced strawberries and allow mixture to cool down a little

5. Fold and top the crêpes with about 1/4 cup each of the strawberry filling (as pictured) or place filling on a flat crêpe and roll up

6. Serve warm and enjoy!

Drink 16oz of water by lunch time

Lunch: Lettuce Combos

Servings: 2

Ingredients:

1 head lettuce

4 tbsp coconut aminos

2 tbsp ginger, grated

1 cup carrots cut into thin strips

8 oz. shitake mushrooms, sliced

1 cup bamboo shots, cut into thin strips

2 cloves garlic

1 tsp fish sauce

Sea salt and black pepper

Procedures:

1. Put skillet over medium heat and put oil
2. Place carrots, garlic, ginger, mushrooms and shoots in skillet and sauté for 2 minutes
3. Add fish sauce and cook for another 5 minutes
4. Remove from heat and set aside
5. Take one lettuce leaf and scoop in the veggie mixture into the lettuce. Wrap into a cone
6. Serve

Drink another 8oz of water after lunch.

Snack: Celery with 2 tablespoons of sunflower butter or baby carrots and few raisins.

Dinner: Slow-cooked Spicy Shredded Beef Tacos and 8oz of water

Ingredients

Taco Ingredients

2 lbs chuck roast

1/4 cup lime juice

3 tbs tomato paste

1/4 cup beef broth

1 medium onion, diced

1 serrano pepper, diced small

1 jalapeno pepper. diced small

3 garlic cloves, minced or pressed

1 tbs chili powder

1 tsp paprika

1/2 tsp cumin

1/2 tsp salt

1/2 tsp pepper

Procedures:

1. Season roast with salt and pepper and set aside

2. Mix dry spices together (chili powder, cumin, paprika) and rub over both sides of roast

3. Place roast in your slow cooker along with the garlic, onion and peppers

4. Combine remaining ingredients (tomato paste, beef stock, lime juice) and pour over beef

5. Cook on Low (8-10 hours) or High (4-6 hours) – meat should be tender and pull apart easily

6. Shred meat with a fork and return to slow cooker. Mix shredded meat with the juices remaining in the slow cooker

7. Make the paleo tortillas or use the shredded beef for a taco salad

8. Top as desired with the avocado cilantro lime sauce

Exercise of the day: 20 minutes Killer Core Workout

As this is a longer workout, it is best that you follow the workout in the video below. Push yourself hard tonight as this is the last workout of the week! Drink plenty of water throughout the exercise.

Workout video → https://www.youtube.com/watch?v=KUjFh4J1dnc

Bedtime: Drink 8oz of water before you go to bed

Day 29 Paleo Challenge

Wake up: Drink water right away. Recommended is 8oz.

Morning workout: Raise your calf with your feet turned out, feet straight and feet turned in. Do this 10 times each.

Breakfast: Coco-Paleo Pancakes and 8oz of water

Yes, you can still have pancakes with the Paleo Diet by using coconut flour on your mixture.

Ingredients:

3tbps. Coconut flour

¼ tsp. baking soda

3 medium-sized eggs

1 tbsp. coconut oil

3 tbsp. coconut milk

2 tbsp. apple sauce (unsweetened)

½ tsp. apple cider vinegar

Procedures:

1. In a bowl, mix the coconut flour and eggs until they are smooth. Add the applesauce, coconut oil, milk, baking soda, vinegar and a small amount of honey.

2. Heat a skillet over medium fire and drizzle hot coconut oil. When the pan is hot, add a small amount of the mixture. Cook the pancakes, until they turn golden brown.

3. Serve with blueberries or strawberries on top and drizzle with honey.

Drink 16oz of water before eating your lunch.

Lunch: Chicken and Avocado Salad Delight

Ingredients:

2 boneless and skinless chicken breasts (cooked and cut into cubes)

1 large avocado (mashed)

2 tbsp. walnuts (chopped)

2 tbsp. fresh cilantro

1 freshly squeezed lime

Salt to taste

Procedures:

1. In a big bowl, combine the cubed chicken and mashed avocado.
2. Throw in the walnuts, finely chopped cilantro, lime juice, and add a pinch of salt to taste.
3. Combine ingredients thoroughly and serve.

Drink another 8oz of water after lunch.

Snack: Homemade Apple Chips

Get a quick sweet fix with these homemade apple chips.

Ingredients:

2 pcs. Honeycrisp apple

1 tsp. cinnamon powder

1 tsp. raw honey

Procedures:

1. Preheat oven to 250°F.

2. Cut the apples in half and remove the seeds. Take a mandolin and slice the apples thinly.

3. Take a baking sheet and lay over with parchment paper.Take the apple slices and lay them separately. Sprinkle the cinnamon powder over the apple slices.

4. Place in the oven and cook or an hour. Flip the apples and cook for another 1 hour. Take out the oven and drizzle with honey.

Consume after cooling or store in an airtight container.

Dinner: Baked Salmon Dinner

This is a simple yet tasty baked salmon recipe.

Ingredients:

1 pc. Wild-caught salmon (32 oz.)

1 lemon (sliced thinly)

1 tbsp. capers

1 tbsp. thyme

Olive oil

Salt and pepper to taste

Procedures:

1. Pre-heat oven to 400°F

2. Prepare a baking sheet and top it with parchment paper. Place the salmon (skin side first) on the sheet and season with salt and pepper.

3. Top the salmon with capers, lemon and fresh thyme and bake in the oven for 25 minutes.

4. Best served, when hot.

Exercise of the day: The Pike

Lie face up with your legs straight, arms at your sides, palms facing down. Raise your legs and torso 45 degrees off the floor. (Your body should look like a "V".) Reach your hands alongside your legs as high as you can without rounding your back.

Start with one set of 8-12 rep. Once you can consistently get 15 reps, add another set.

Bedtime: Drink 16oz of water before you go to bed

Day 30 Paleo Challenge

Wake up: Drink water right away. Recommended is 8oz.

Morning workout: Do 10 push-ups to get your blood flowing

Breakfast: 8oz of water and Heavenly Ham n' Eggs

A simple two-ingredient recipe you'll want to eat, every morning!

Ingredients:

4 slices of ham

2 eggs

(spices for flavor)

Procedures:

1. Preheat your oven to 400 °F

2. Prepare a muffin pan by greasing it with coconut oil.

3. Place two pieces of ham on top of each other in one muffin cup. Repeat with the next muffin cup.

4. Crack the egg on top of the ham

    a. *(Optional: add scallions, basil, etc. on your egg for more flavor)*

5. Bake for 15 minutes and serve.

Drink 16oz of water before eating your lunch.

Lunch: Veggie-bun Sandwich

Ingredients:

1 pc. red bell pepper

2 slices turkey ham

½ avocado (cut into strips)

1 pc. seaweed strips

Procedures:

1. Take the bell pepper and slice it in half and remove the seeds.
2. Take one piece of bell pepper and top it with the ham, seaweed, and avocado.
3. Top with the other half of the bell pepper and stick a toothpick in the center.
4. Enjoy.

Drink another 8oz of water after lunch.

Snack: Celery with 2 tablespoons of sunflower butter or baby carrots and few raisins.

Dinner: Low-carb Paleo Patties and 8oz of water

Ingredients:

16 oz. ground lean turkey

1 tsp. Paprika

½ tsp. coriander

1 tsp. powdered onion

a pinch of cayenne pepper

a pinch of salt

a pinch of ground pepper

2 pcs. green onions (chopped)

1 pc. tomato (sliced)

2 cups arugula

1 pc. avocado (sliced)

Procedures:

1. In a bowl, place the ground turkey and add the onion powder, salt, pepper, paprika, cayenne pepper, and green onions and combine everything.

2. Use your hands to form into burger patties.

3. Heat the grill and cook the burgers for 5 minutes, per side.

4. Place the cooked patties over the arugula, tomatoes, and avocado. Serve.

Exercise of the day: Tree-pose Yoga

This pose will have your abdominals working overtime to help you stay grounded on one leg.

Shift your weight onto your left foot. Draw your right knee into your chest, grab your ankle, and press the bottom of your right foot onto your left thigh. If you feel wobbly, keep your hand on your ankle while it is pressed into your thigh. If you're finding your balance easily, press your palms together in front of your chest. Brace your abdominals in tight to your spine, making sure you can still breathe easily. Find a focal point and focus your gaze while you hold the pose for 10 long, deep breaths. Repeat on the other leg.

Bedtime: Drink 8oz of water before you go to bed

Chapter 7: Paleo Diet for Sportsmen

When the concept of Paleo diet was brought forward (the idea of retracing our ancestor's dietary plans such as intake of vegetables, high proteins and fresh fruits in abundance), the idea received massive attention from nutritional and medical communities. Some nutritionists even termed it as the best nutritious diet available on planet Earth. Today, most sports coaches recommend Paleo diet to their respective team members. The reason being:

- Typical diet for sportsmen (refined sugars, starches and concentrated with grains) is detrimental to the athlete's health, performance, and recovery

- The acid-base and glycemic load balance affect the sportsman's performance

- The consumption of simple sugars and starches only benefits the sportsman during the immediate period of post-exercise. They do not have long-term benefits.

Fortunately, Paleo diet for sportsmen has the effect of maximizing the athlete's performance irrespective of the completion level or sports endurance range.

You're a power athlete, regardless of the sport you compete in, for example, rugby or football. Therefore, you should have the ability to fuel accordingly. Endurance athletes who are also cross fitters are an exception. The needs of power athletes are different compared to endurance athletes or couch potatoes, and they should tweak Paleo diet to their specific needs.

Whether you want to add bulk, maintain your current strength and muscle mass, or lean out, how you eat or your dietary approach is what will matter. Robb Wolf, The Paleo Solution author, suggests that people in a weight cutting endeavor should eat considerable quantities of bodyweight as follows each day: protein (1-1.25g), calories (15-17g), carbs (50-100g), and some healthy fats. For a female with a weight of 150-pound, her intake should comprise proteins (150-187g), calories (2250-2550), carbs (50-100g) and fat (close to 155-160g).

Robb Wolf recommends a post-workout starchy carbs intake and relatively low carb consumption. If possible, you can enhance your loss of fat by taking branched-chain amino acids of 10-20g while training, if you want to maintain your muscle strength and body size. As an athlete, eating calories whose largest percentage comes from carbs during the period of post-workout is a wise idea.

However, for an athlete to build his muscle, it requires more than good nutrition. An athlete needs to have ample sleeping time, as well as train very hard. This is because building body muscle requires a person to eat more and if no caution is being put into consideration, the athlete might end up gaining weight, instead of improving muscle strength. For hypertrophy, the right environment has to be created by the athlete, by ensuring that the recovery and training are on point.

The precise prescriptions given below should be simple to follow and adhered to strictly by the athlete. The dietary plan is to help an athlete remain true to his Paleo diet. Paleo diet comprises of breakfast, snacks, lunch and even evening meals which are suitable for any athlete who has a goal of improving his performance and overall health.

Power Athlete Dietary Plan

Breakfast

(between 5:30-6:30 AM)

This is the suitable time to take a pre-workout breakfast; baked yam whizzed with almond butter, protein powder (egg white), green tea (natural decaf) and a banana. At around 6:30 AM, you can take a trainer-carbohydrate gel.

(between 9:30-10:00 AM)

You can take a quick recovery drink for the post-workout. Alternatively, consider taking glucose, protein powder (egg white) and cantaloupe. Moreover, keep yourself hydrated-drink water frequently.

For continuity of the body recovery, preparation for future sessions and the restoration of body alkalinity, consider taking raisins.

Lunch

(11:30-12:00 PM)

As an athlete, the best meals to consume at this time include grilled chicken breast, flaxseed oil, an apple and flash-sauteed asparagus.

Afternoon meal

(3:00 PM)

Chopped egg whites and applesauce that is natural unsweetened.

(4:30 PM)

The athlete can take carbohydrate gel as post-workout recovery diet. Being a high glycemic fruit, a banana is also significant in the recovery process.

Dinner

At this time, the athlete can eat steamed kale, avocado, sliced oranges, poached wild salmon, fresh lime juice, mixed green salad, sliced strawberries and extra virgin oil.

Endurance Athlete Dietary Plan

During an off-day from training, an endurance athlete can choose to follow this dietary plan:

Breakfast

Fresh strawberries and blueberries, sautéed spinach (with olive oil or garlic) and barramundi, or poached cod are good as first meals for an endurance athlete.

Alternatively, the athlete can consider taking chopped egg whites, flax seed oil, steamed broccoli and sliced orange.

Lunch

During lunch hours, eat grapes, grilled chicken, lime wedge, avocado and olive oil.

Afternoon meal

An afternoon meal is supposed to be light for a person to be active throughout the day. The best meals for an afternoon include sliced pear, lean turkey breast, raw almond butter and mache lettuce.

Dinner

The list of ingredients for an endurance athlete dinner meal include lime wedge and walnut oil, grilled green onion, tomato with spinach salad, red onions, kangaroo kebabs-lean meat, yellow bell peppers, lemon juice and olive oil.

Snack

Green decaf tea or herbal tea, cinnamon, an apple, lemon juice. Lemon juice, in this case, prevents oxidation or browning.

By taking a close observation of the ingredients of the different meals given above, you'll notice that the Paleolithic diet is simply a throwback dietary plan similar to that of the caveman days. It advocates eating fresh vegetables, healthy fats, fresh fruits and lean proteins. Paleo diet is perfect for athletes since it lacks starches, processed sugars, and grains.

Case study:

In 2004, Nell Stephenson (during Ironman race) contracted a parasite. Despite following the prescribed medication, her health deteriorated for months. She developed stomach problems and gluten-intolerance, yet she ate healthy foods, at all times. Tired of her typical diet, Stephenson decided to try a different diet and see if her health would improve.

She decided to go, the Paleo way. A diet plan which dates back to caveman era before Agricultural revolution. After three days, Stephenson had already experienced significant improvements in her overall health. As a result, Stephenson decided to start a blog called "Paleoista" and even wrote a book particularly on Paleo diet to enlighten dieters who live in the "dark."

The popularity of Paleo has seen tremendous growth in society. However, the basic tenets of Paleo seemingly counter to the endurance athletes and runners traditional carbo-loading. That is because Paleo diet avoids dairy, processed foods, legumes, grains and grains, as mentioned earlier.

While a majority of the athletes supposedly eat fresh vegetables and fruits and lean proteins (or, at least, try), many people still eat more starches, processed sugars, and grains.

Restrictive Diet

With simple little adjustments, the benefits which an athlete accrues from Paleo menus are many. As a result of its micronutrient content, Paleo provides a better and long-term recovery compared to sugar and high-starch diet. Moreover, Paleo enables an athlete to attend to training without any stress.

Dividing the diet of an athlete into three stages is vital. A Paleo diet should form the basis of an athlete's meals! However, immediately after, before and during workouts, several adjustments to the diet could be needed.

About two hours before a hard workout session or a long race, the athlete should consider eating meals which have low fiber content and moderate glycemic index.

When there is an extended race or athletic event, a majority of the athletes will require sports gels or drinks, which are forms of quickly-processed carbohydrates. Even the athletes whose diets are 100% Paleo acknowledge that they need these carbohydrates gels in times of ultramarathons or when they are competing in Ironman races. But if the athletic event is short and spans for a few minutes, water is good enough.

Blood sugar fluctuations are leveled out more efficiently whenever an athlete utilizes more of the stored fats with their working muscles when the athlete concentrates on diets which have low carbohydrates. This body change is reportedly experienced by athletes who adopt the Paleo way of dieting after about six weeks. Other people may experience the changes earlier or a bit later.

Immediately after long or intense workouts, the protein and carbohydrates recovery drink intake by an athlete should be in the ration 5:4. Moreover, significant muscle rebuilding and recovery can be ensured after a workout if the athlete engages in short window eating.

Imaginary Perfect Diet

The best times to possibly go non-Paleo and focus on carbohydrates for an athlete is during the time immediately after hard workouts or exercise. At this period, pasta and bagels are examples of starchy foods which an athlete can eat. They contain high glucose which is paramount for recovery. Other alternatives include potatoes, raisin, and yams.

Most athletes who find Paleo diet to be inefficient or ineffective is because they either not plan, not assess their bodies or not understand the Paleo diet. Most importantly, calorie restrictions or low-calories intake is not what Paleo is all about- a common mistake made by most athletes.

In some cases, you'll find athletes who have adopted Paleo, but for sustained endurance, they still have challenges eating appropriately even after months of trials. Such athletes focus on dates, potatoes and applesauce for energy, but if the training is intense, the athlete "should hit plenty of dates".

Appropriate planning of your possible food intake requires more work than you think. However, if the athlete had nurtured a habit of eating foods close to Paleo and relatively healthy, except for legume and grains, the changes would be minimal or even unnoticeable. Paleo, especially for athletes who depend on sports nutrition bars and electrolyte drinks but eat no vegetables, forms a healthy diet structure.

A Paleo diet, more importantly, carries the following guarantees to an athlete:

- ✓ More vitamins
- ✓ More antioxidants
- ✓ Increased fat oxidation
- ✓ Better retained muscles
- ✓ Recovery of muscles

All these improves an athlete's running speed by: strengthening his immune system, improving his long-event endurance and balancing his pH levels. With Paleo, an athlete's body begins functioning optimally.

Athlete's Paleo Diet Guide

Today, people have tremendously embraced the consumption of optimal foods; courtesy of the recommendations by nutritionists and other medical experts. Optimal foods encompass a lean animal protein, fruits, and vegetables. The promise that these foods meet a dieter's nutritional needs is perhaps the reason most people have adapted to them. Thrive by eating these or compromise your performance and health by strictly limiting or avoiding them.

However, with respect to the time immediately after, before or during workouts, serious athletes need to bend the Paleo diet rules a bit. This is because a lot of demands are placed on the body, which was not common in the stone age period. The unique demands of serious athletes include prolonged time of sustained output of high energy and quick recovery need. Therefore, the athlete has to have some latitude to consume foods which are non-optimal but under a certain limit.

The following five periods best explains these exceptions:

Period 1: Eating before Exercise

In brief, an athlete is recommended to eat, at least 2-3 hours before any long race or hard workout, foods containing carbohydrates of moderate or low glycemic index. At this point, proteins and fat can still be eaten. However, the food must have low fiber content. Moreover, for every hour remaining before the race or workout, an athlete should eat 200-300 calories, if possible.

Period 2: Eating while in Exercise

Carbohydrates of high glycemic index and that are in fluids form are the best foods during races, hard or long workout sessions for serious athletes. However, the choice of sports drinks depends on the athlete's taste and preference. However, for events that last only an hour or few minutes long such as warm-ups, the athlete doesn't necessarily have to take any carbohydrates. According to your experience, the exercise nature or body size modification, per hour intake of 200-400 calories can be your starting point. The point is, increase your calories intake with an increase in the event's duration.

Period 3: Eating Immediately After

In the post workout or post race minutes (say 30 minutes; after a highly intense or prolonged exercise or long workout), an athlete should take protein and carbohydrate recovery drinks which contain both nutrients in the ratio 5:4 respectively.

Alternatively, an athlete can make a Paleo smoothie for recovery purposes by blending; banana with fruit juice ounces, glucose tablespoons (3 to 5), whey sources/egg protein powder (3 tbsp.) and salt (2 pinches). After a race or hard workout, this recovery smoothie should be every athlete's highest priority.

Period 4: Extended Recovery Eating

Hours after a run or intensive workout, the athlete can continue concentrating on carbohydrate diet (carbs of a high or moderate load of glycemic) along with protein, keeping the carb-protein 4:5 ratio in mind. During this time, non-optimal foods, for example, glucose, pasta, corn, bread, rice, and bagels can be eaten. These foods are significant contributors to the recovery process. However, the most suitable foods for this period include yams, raisins, sweet potatoes and potatoes.

Period 5: LongTerm Eating

LongTerm eating simply refers to eating before the athlete starts a new workout in the next session. During LongTerm eating, the athlete should retrace his Paleo diet schedule- eat optimal foods as this helps to boost the athlete's general performance.

The Recommended Fat, Carbs and Protein Intake Quantity

The Paleo diet doesn't provide any parameters or limits of the Fat, Carbs, and Protein Intake Quantity! However, it advocates an optimal quantity intake. However, what quantity is optimal quantity? Well, the macronutrient requirement of a dieter changes according to the demand. An athlete should periodize along with training or exercise session. All year round, a serious athlete should maintain a consistent and strict protein intake. For calories intake, an athlete should maintain a 20-25% range. Compared to our stone age ancestors consumption range, this intake is at the low end because of the increased carbohydrate intake by an athlete in Period 1 to 4 which has the effect of diluting protein.

On the other hand, as the seasons of training change, diet periodization produces opposing and significant swings in regards to the athlete's carbohydrate intake and fat intake. During the general/base preparation time, there is a decrease in carbohydrate intake as the diet takes a shift for increased fat intake. At this point, more healthy fat should be consumed since the utilization of body fat is the training's primary objective. Calories stand at 30% while carbohydrates stand at 50%.

During the particular preparation time (peak and build period), the body experiences greater demand as the training increases intensity for fuel exercise. It's at this latter time that Period 3 and Period 4 become more crucial and critical on the recovery of the athlete. At this point, fat and calories intake drop to about 20%, whereas carbohydrate intake rises to about 60%.

During the transition, tapering or peaking period when there is minimal training, the caloric intake should be significantly reduced or limited, to avoid excessive or undesired weight gain.

Importance of Paleo Diet to Athletes

A person's fitness and health are not synonymous. Unfortunately, a majority of the athletes are only fit, but not healthy. The performance potential is greatly reduced by frequent overtraining, injury or illness. The Paleo diet makes significant improvements to an athlete's health. Here's how:

> ➤ The branched-chain amino acids intake enhance anabolic function and muscle development. In endurance athletes, immunosuppression is also counteracted.

> ➤ Healing is promoted, and tissue inflammation is reduced due to the changes in the omega-3 and omega-6 ratio. Hence, this prevents asthmatic conditions.

> ➤ The body acidity and acidosis catabolic effect on muscles and bone are reduced and this is known as an anti-aging benefit.

➢ Increased trace nutrients for the recovery process.

Conclusion

Congratulations on completing the 30-Day Paleo Challenge! I hope this book was able to help you to learn about the things you need to know in following the Paleo Diet and living the Paleo life. Many people have already seen the benefits of the diet, and it's time that you gain these benefits too!

Do note that the above are a guide to help you get started. Feel free to change the routines according to your endurance level. If you follow the tips and try the recipes I shared with you, I assure you that you will see a better and healthier You!

Again, thank you for downloading this book! Spread the good news and enjoy the Paleo Lifestyle today!

Finally, if you've received value from this book, please take the time to share your thoughts and post a review on Amazon. It'd be greatly appreciated!

Thank you and good luck!

Check Out These Other Books

Below you'll find some of my best-selling books that are popular on Amazon and Kindle as well. Simply go to Amazon and search for these titles under my Author name.

Diabetes Diet: Ultimate Diabetic Cookbook - Top Most Delicious Recipes to Help You Get Started on Diabetes Diet

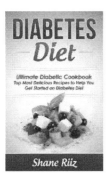

It's a hard blow to find out you have diabetes or even pre-diabetes. When you hear your doctor explain the challenges you're facing, you know your life will never be the same again. One of the changes you probably need to make is the foods you choose to eat. Adopting a diabetic diet is the surest way to get your diabetes under control and start feeling better again.

So, what is a diabetes diet? The main feature of this type of diet is that you need to eat fewer carbohydrates. In fact, many diabetics are encouraged to follow a plan called "carb counting." When you count carbs, you simply add up the carbohydrate servings each time you eat and don't exceed a certain number of servings based on your caloric needs.

While carb counting is effective in reducing the amount of sugar in your bloodstream, many people find that it isn't enough. About 8 to 12 hours after you've eaten a meal loaded with excessive amounts of unhealthy fats, your blood sugar tends to rise significantly. So, for most people, it's also important to limit fat servings.

21-Day Weight Loss Challenge – How to Lose 15 Pounds with Low Carb Diet

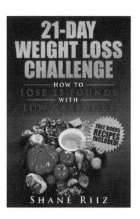

Low carb diets are your best bet to win the battle for weight control. Healthy eating is one of the strongest foundations to achieve not only weight loss but also total health and wellness. A properly balanced diet, combined with other positive health decision, will result in vast improvements in your health and lifestyle.

When you have a proper diet that takes into account all nutrients you need, from proteins, healthy fats, minerals, vitamins and carbs, then you are one step closer toward achieving your health goals. Diet serves as the fuel to power all your body tissues and organs to maintain its optimum performance. The better your diet is, the better fuel your body can use. Of particular importance is the carb component of your diet.

Carbs & Weight Control

The low carb diet works because it zeroes in on one of the primary causes of weight gain, the accumulation of fats. The link between carbs and weight gain is found between the transformation of carbs into calories and then into fats. Carbs are meant to power your body throughout the day. When it is consumed, it becomes calories, which is the actual fuel needed by the body to meet your demands. However, when you consume too many calories, and your body does not utilize them, for example in a sedentary lifestyle, calories are stored as fats.

And this is where the weight control problem becomes apparent. The more carbs you consume and the less activity you do, the more fats are stored, and the more weight is gained. When you have low carb consumption, there is less amount of fats to be stored; sometimes you can even consume and expend the exact amount of calories you need for the day.

The Migraine Cure: Causes of Migraine and the Ultimate Solutions to Relief Your Migraine for Life

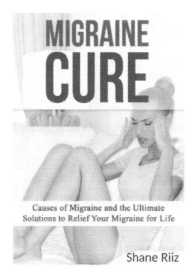

What is a migraine? Everyone, at least once in their life, has confronted with a terrible headache that often tended to reappear. It is a public health issue of substantial impact on both the sufferer and society.

To clear your doubt, migraine is defined as a chronic neurological disorder characterized by repetitive mild to intense headaches, frequently in association with some neurological symptoms. It may appear only once every few years or several times a week. It can last for a couple of hours and three days. The pain begins in the first part of the day, on one-half of the head. (Actually, the word "migraine" is borrowed from a Greek word that means "half-head.") Rarely, the entire head is filled up with pain.

Associated symptoms might include vomiting, nausea, photophobia, sonophobia, or osmophobia. The pain usually gets worse by physical activity. More than one-third of people with migraine headaches sense an aura: a temporary visual, language, sensory or motor interference which indicates that a headache will soon appear. Sometimes an aura can come with brief or no problem succeeding it.

Migraines are considered to be caused by a combination of environmental and inheritable factors. Modifying hormone levels might play a role too, as migraines have more slightly effect on boys than girls before pubescence, but about three times more on women than men. The threat of migraines usually diminishes during pregnancy. The precise mechanisms of a migraine are unknown. It is, although, believed to be a neurovascular condition. The leading theory is associated with the intensification regarding excitability of the cerebral cortex and variable control of pain neurons within the trigeminal nucleus belonging to the brainstem.

PALEO DIET: ULTIMATE PALEO COOKBOOK FOR EFFECTIVE WEIGHT LOSS AND HEALTHY LIVING WITH DELICIOUS PALEO RECIPES

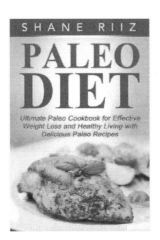

The Paleo diet is one the few diets that is gradually gaining worldwide acceptance. Its success can be credited to its unique take on the proper diet that is best for consumption. The basic foundation of the diet is found in the Paleolithic era or most commonly known as the Stone Age. The idea behind the diet is that our human ancestors, the cavemen, are one of the most physically fit humans to have every walked the face of the earth. The secret behind the cavemen's ability is their source of nutrients and energy.

During those ancient times, the caveman diet consisted primarily of all natural foods. The food was neither processed nor refined. The contents of the diet were also low on sugar and dairy. The major food groups, which were also the only ones available at that time, were those that were naturally growing in the environment of the caveman. These were simple meats, vegetables, fruits, nuts, and seeds.

Fast forward to our modern time; our food options are now littered with some of the unhealthiest food in history. High cholesterol fast foods, high sugar content sweets, high sodium preserved foods and other refined and processed foods make up the daily intake of people today. The problem is despite these changes in our food options; our genetic make-up remains the same as with our cavemen ancestors. These means our dietary needs remain the same.

Another problem with the food options today is that even if you buy meats, vegetables, or fruits in the hope that they will be similar to the caveman's own food options, it will rarely be the case. For example, while meat before was grass-fed, today artificial feeds and chemicals are fed or injected to cows, pigs, chicken, fish and other sources of food. While vegetables grew using the natural nutrients of the soil and earth, today there are grown using fertilizers and protected using pesticides.

The solution that the Paleo diet offers are simple, to achieve the same health, endurance and overall well-being of the cavemen, we need to choose only food items that bear the closest resemblance to their diet. This means grass-fed meats, organic vegetables and fruits and other healthier options. It is fortunate that these specialty products are becoming more and more available to the average consumer.

Although the term Paleo diet can be credited to Walter Voegtin, a doctor, and gastroenterologist in 1975, it was Joseph Knowles in 1913, who first presented the idea of the benefits of an all natural diet. By immersing himself in the hunger and gatherer lifestyle for 2 whole months, he emerged with a better health and a stronger body.

Claim Your FREE Bonus!

As a token of appreciation for buying my book, I would like to give away a FREE e-book, *"SUGAR DETOX: Easy Guide to Cure Sugar Addictions, Stop Sugar Cravings and Lose Weight with Sugar Detox."*

May you gain more valuable insights in achieving your weight loss goals!

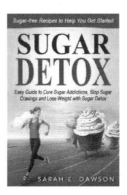

Plus, by signing up to our subscription, you will also receive <u>FREE KINDLE BOOKS,</u> <u>recipes, tips and tools</u> to help you attained the weight and health you desire.

See you on the inside!

To claim your FREE bonus, go to the URL below:

http://bit.ly/sugar_detox_ebook

52315303R00094